PSYCHOLOGICAL
ASPECTS
of the
CARE
of
HOSPITALIZED
PATIENTS

EDITION 4

PSYCHOLOGICAL ASPECTS of the CARE of HOSPITALIZED PATIENTS

EDITION 4

Lisa Robinson, R.N., Ph.D., F.A.A.N., C.S.

Professor, Psychiatric Nursing
School of Nursing
University of Maryland
Baltimore, Maryland

F.A. DAVIS COMPANY ⬦ Philadelphia

Library of Congress Cataloging in Publication Data

Robinson, Lisa, R.N.
  Psychological aspects of the care of hospitalized patients.

  Includes bibliographies and index.
  1. Nurse and patient.   2. Nursing—psychological aspects.
3. Hospital patients—Psychology. I. Title.
RT86.3.R63 1984   610.73'3   83-20972
ISBN 0-8036-7473-2

For Karen,
on the occasion
of her becoming a nurse.

Foreword

"Wherever there is a heart and an intellect, the diseases of the physical frame are tinged with the peculiarities of these . . . So Roger Chillingworth—the man of skill, the kind and friendly physician—strove to go deep into his patient's bosom . . . probing everything with a cautious touch. . . ." If the doctor can ". . . bring his mind into such affinity with his patient's, that this last shall unawares have spoken what he imagines himself only to have thought; if such revelations be received without tumult, and acknowledged not so often by an uttered sympathy as by silence, an inarticulate breath, and here and there a word, to indicate that all is understood; if to these qualifications of a confidant be joined the advantages afforded by his recognized character as a physician—then, at some inevitable moment, will the soul of the sufferer be dissolved, and flow forth in a dark, but transparent stream, bringing all its mysteries into the daylight."

These words were written around 1850 by Nathaniel Hawthorne and are contained in *The Scarlet Letter*. They recognize what patients and poets have known intuitively from the beginning, but what professional clinicians, unfortunately, must be taught.

The training of doctors and nurses includes a series of landmark experiences, all of which are potentially overwhelming. The first encounter with a cadaver; the first autopsy—in which the body is now linked systematically with the story of a recently living person (who could not be saved by medical science); the first diseased, suffering, hopelessly dependent, dying patient—all these meetings with man's ultimate nakedness before natural forces evoke anxiety and the building of a suit of defensive armor. The armor is necessary if the clinician is to be useful to the patient. It is necessary for the achievement of what has been called *detached concern*. Detached concern means reducing the likelihood that the clinician's own fears about death and disease will give him or her trouble as decisions must be made about what to do with sick or dying patients. It means an intelligent awareness of what is happening without the kind of emotional involvement that interferes with one's judgment. It means relative freedom from the tendency to identify oneself with a patient who, without the clinician's realizing it, may have come to represent his own parent or sibling or spouse or child.

On the other hand, the clinician or therapist, from whatever professional discipline, will not succeed in his tasks if the patient is viewed as an object, a specimen, or laboratory material with no needs or feelings of its own. And a tendency to view the patient this way is part of the emotional suit of armor that the future practitioner begins to acquire at the very onset of his career as a student. It is for this reason that students of nursing and medicine, the two health professions that involve most intimate contact with other human beings who hurt and fear, require deliberate attention during their professional education to their own feelings and attitudes. It was for this reason that Dr. Francis Peabody of Harvard, one of the fathers of medical practice in this country, found it necessary to state that "the secret of the care *of* the patient is to care *for* the patient."

Now, let's not discuss clinicians in general, but nurses in particular. The physician is mobile; he may see patients in several hospitals, confining himself from the impact of feelings by focusing his attention on the scientific aspects of the case before him. He is usually not present at mealtime, at toilet time, or at sleep time, when the human needs of the person temporarily transformed into a patient demand recognition. The people who are *there* are the nurses and, increasingly, their aides. And what do they encounter?

The author expertly delineates the fear, depression, dependency, and deprivation-induced disorientation of persons incarcerated in the alien hospital cage. She notes, too, their anger and sometimes chaotic attempts to escape or make contact with others. Perhaps a central, unifying theme, present in all humans contemplating dissolution, is that of loneliness. This is superimposed—by loss of function, bodily disintegration, and separation from the familiar—upon something already present: what Kierkegaard called the "shut-upness" of civilized men today. At its extreme is what Binswanger termed "naked existence" and what Harry Stack Sullivan considered part of the development of psychotic states: ". . . A schizophrenic patient at St. Elizabeth's Hospital in Washington, D.C., writing under the pen name of Ethne Tabor, published a poem called "Panic" in 1950. Here is isolation starkly defined:

> And is there anyone at all
> And is there anyone at all?
> And does this empty silence have to be?
> And is there no one there at all
> To answer me?

Loneliness, it seems to me, is at the core of what the hospital nurse encounters. It is not always obvious, for we are all well schooled in the concealment of feeling, even from ourselves. But it is there in the person trapped in his failing body, vulnerable to death and strangers and the surging fears and memories stored from earliest weak, dependent childhood. It demands communication, at least a moment of shared contact. How possible this is is problematic. Sympathy is easy, but it is not the same thing. As Albert Camus wrote, sympathy is "a board chairman's emotion; it comes cheap after catastrophes." Other words have been used in an attempt to distill the essence of human contact: empathy, congruence, identification, mutual awareness, the intrusion of one into the private world of another. Edith Weigert wrote of the "rediscovery of trust" as a therapeutic turning point. Sonneman regarded as prerequisite "an unconditional readiness to recognize the other and share his world with him . . . [an] openness of the inner horizon. . . ."

The author is more modest in her goals. By means of this book she hopes to assist the nurse in initiating communication with the patient. She provides a frame of reference that will make disparate behavioral events become coherent. Her guidelines will permit the nurse to organize her own behavior and feelings and, perhaps, give her the security to realize some of her own latent capacities for therapeutic contact with others. One can ask for no more.

EUGENE B. BRODY, M.D.
Director, Institute of Psychiatry
and Human Behavior
University of Maryland School
of Medicine

Preface

It is extremely difficult to rewrite and add to several editions of a book, because one's interests, types of life experience, and maturity change, as do the needs of the book's audience. All of these factors have influenced the fourth edition of *Psychological Aspects of the Care of Hospitalized Patients*.

I am mindful, as well as appreciative, of the original book's reception. I believed then as now that this response from readers reflects the timeliness of the topic and the style in which the book is written. I have wanted to preserve the style as well as the book's focus. To this end, the topics in the new edition remain largely the same, although current issues of concern to caregivers are reflected in contributions by Dr. Kenneth Solomon on the geriatric patient, and by Dr. Mary Ann Walsh Eells on the alcoholic patient. I have added material on the chronically ill patient and the special patient. The chapter on the special patient may be confusing to readers of the previous editions, who may note another chapter by the same title. In more recent rumination, I decided that the previously titled chapter really concerned itself with only one type of special patient, that is, the health care provider as patient. Therefore, I have retitled that chapter to reflect its content. The new chapter, entitled The Special Patient, focuses on a broader group of individuals who cause disruptions of the normal functioning of hospital systems by their explicit or subtle demands for attention.

The new edition of this book reflects a trend toward specialization. While I did not plan a modification away from the generalist's interests (with its behavioral orientation), current foci of the health care delivery system seem to dictate the need for content in these added areas and in other areas not yet included.

It is no longer possible to write in exactly the same style that I wrote in 14 years ago, because I have changed. While I have tried to preserve those elements of simplicity, straightforwardness, and descriptiveness that characterized the first three editions, I recognize that my own writing style is different. I have tried to maintain a balance between the old and new qualities in the writing. Where I have failed, I apologize in advance; where I have succeeded, I am grateful to patients and students who have given me clinical material from which to draw.

For the sake of clarity, the feminine gender, third-person pronoun usually refers to the nurse, the masculine pronoun to the patient. This is not to be construed as a bias of mine. It is merely an expediency. I am cognizant of the fine contribution of male nurses and of the abundance of female patients.

My own clinical experiences as well as entry into the midlife decade have made me more sensitive to the issues confronting adults who have weathered the child-bearing years and who now face return to full-time employment or the disillusionment of unachieved goals. It is in these years that human beings begin to experience physical decline, chronic illness, or at least irreversibility of bodily deterioration. Some integrate this phase of aging, while others look to panaceas such as health spas, new careers or mates, and alcohol. We observe the tribulations of our parents and relatives and hope that our own will be traversed more easily. The new edition is, in part, about these issues.

I hope that this edition will contribute to the scope of nursing practice and help to make us more sensitive to, more gentle with, and more tolerant of others as they undergo the hardships they must endure. If we nurture human beings and help them to regain their health or help them to accept what they must, I shall feel satisfied with this volume's usefulness to health care providers.

LR

Contributors

Mary Ann Walsh Eells, Ed.D., R.N., C.N.

Associate Professor
University of Maryland
School of Nursing
Baltimore, Maryland

Kenneth Solomon, M.D.

Adjunct Assistant Professor
Department of Psychiatry
University of Maryland
School of Medicine
Baltimore, Maryland

Associate Director
Education and Planning
Levindale Hebrew Geriatric Center and Hospital
Baltimore, Maryland

Contents

1
Introduction

Lisa Robinson, R.N., Ph.D., F.A.A.N., C.S.

The general hospital is an institution providing health services which include diagnostic tests, medical treatment, surgical intervention, and rehabilitative care. In the past, hospital regimen was directed to the physical needs of patients; more recently, attention has also been focused on their emotional needs.

Each person who is admitted to a general hospital brings with him not only a physical illness but also a definitive mental set that will influence both the manner in which he assumes his role as a *patient* and the course of his hospitalization. The manner in which a sick person responds as a patient will also be influenced by the person's illness, the route of admission to the hospital, his fantasies about the institution and the people in it, and his fantasies concerning himself and the problem making hospitalization necessary. Information that the individual has acquired indirectly or facts that have been told him by acquaintances and his doctor will also have some bearing on his interpretation of the patient role.

The individual contemplating admission to a hospital will cope with the stress of his hospitalization in the same manner that he would cope with other major stresses in his life. The mechanisms he has become accustomed to using to buffer himself against other anxieties and external dangers will also be used to help fend off the uncomfortable feelings that overwhelm him as he faces illness and hospitalization.

If the stressed person has always tended to adhere to strict schedules, he will probably seem markedly conscious of time and regimen during his hospitalization. If the potential patient has been known to be a colorful person, prone to an intense show of feelings and unusual preoccupation with his own reactions, he is likely to demonstrate such behavior in the hospital. This person will probably be far more uncomfortable than a normally serene person would be when reports of tests or progress are very detailed and explicit.[1] This is the kind of person who is liable to entertain extreme fantasies concerning each new symptom. The person with these personality traits has a rich inner life and the type of intellect that can magnify minor signs and symptoms into ones of major proportions. Such a process is prompted by anxiety.[2]

All persons live under stress. Eustress, or normal stress, as described by Selye, differs from distress in that it is necessary for maintenance of the healthy individual's productive functioning. Distress occurs when the degree of stress is greater than that which the individual can handle in normal functioning. Illness, hospitalization, and treatment are usually challenging to the individual and are sources of stress. To maintain the dynamic equilibrium of both psyche and soma, the patient calls upon additional coping behaviors and defenses against anxiety. Current nursing studies indicate that people use protective styles of coping that are related to their personality types and perhaps to their orientation to locus of control.[3]

The character of the person's illness will influence his course of hospitalization. If the disease process is not diagnosed, the patient is likely to feel quite anxious. If the illness is minor, the patient may regard his hospitalization as an annoyance and a situation to be simply tolerated. Patients convalescing from heart attacks often feel this way because they do not feel sick.

Some people hospitalized for terminal illness will show no apparent appropriate reaction. This is often a demonstration of the mechanism of denial being effectively used.

People who enter the hospital through the emergency room tend to have more difficulty with adjustment than those who can plan their admissions and begin to call upon successful defense mechanisms and coping behaviors prior to the actual hospitalization.

Fantasies concerning hospitals will markedly influence a patient's course of hospitalization. Almost all pediatric nurses have witnessed the abysmal results when a well-meaning mother tells her child before he goes to the operating room that he is going to get his hair cut, or that he is going to a party, or some other contrived tale. On the other hand, some patients enter the hospital expecting harsh, painful treatment and an absence of humaneness. As these patients correct their fantasies by seeing and hearing what hospitals are really like, they tend to relax and adjust more comfortably to hospitalization.

Most people enter the hospital with an array of fantasies concerning their lack of power, their hopelessness, and their helplessness. Some patients fantasize about their omnipotence. This type of thinking is often a defensive maneuver designed to protect the individual against overwhelming fear or feelings of helplessness.

Patients have similar fantasies about the people who care for them. Caregiving personnel may be experienced as nurturing agents or as authoritative and cruel people. They can be perceived as playing numerous roles, depending on the patient's perceptions and his background experiences. Patients sometimes have fantasies about the motives of the nurses and doctors; at times they question the situations that gratify hospital personnel.

Some of the fantasies are conscious; some are not. Some fantasies become conscious during hospitalization; others never do. The fantasy material that comes into the patient's awareness will often be modified as he encounters the realities of his hospitalization. Those fantasies that do not become conscious to the patient will nonetheless influence his response to hospitalization.[4,5]

Childhood experiences play a major role in the individual's interpretation of the patient role and his reaction to the hospital staff. If the sick person has had warm, comfortable experiences with kind, loving parents, he is likely to accept his doctor and nurses as reasonable authority figures who are concerned with his well-being. If his childhood experiences have led him to expect parental figures to be punitive or sadistic, the sick individual is likely to view his nurses and doctor in a similar way. Whether the person is able to follow his treatment regimen or is uncooperative, whether he is anxious or demanding, or whether he is inflexible or suspicious will all be predetermined by his life experiences.

Nurses come to their jobs with a mental set influenced by their fantasies and expectations also. Their responses to patients and nursing problems are influenced by their needs and their cultural and psychological backgrounds. The men and women who decide to become nurses arrive at their choice of profession by a very deliberate set of steps. Their childhood upbringing and prior education have influenced the professional choice. Living experiences have led them to believe that nursing would be gratifying work. Sometimes certain deficits in individuals' lives have made them more aware of the desire to care for others.

Nurses sometimes view themselves as mothering, nurturing people; some care for sick people in an unconscious effort to acquire for themselves the care they were deprived of in childhood. Nurses tend to expect their patients to be passive recipients of nursing ministrations. The good patient is one who is quiet, cooperative, and uncomplaining. He is a patient who accepts without question the nursing care offered to him.

Nurses respond to patients' needs and demands in accordance with the message they receive concerning the patients' desires, the ability they have to provide for the patients' needs, and their evaluation of the validity of the patients' needs. The nurse who was raised in a family where emotional outbursts were considered to be in poor taste will probably find it difficult to respond in a positive manner to the patient who cries loudly and often. On the other hand, the same nurse may work ideally with an emotionally undemonstrative patient, because this nurse can respond in a realistic and appropriate way to the patient.

Sometimes patients do not meet the expectations of nurses. At times, nurses do not meet the expectations of patients. In these instances, nursing problems are likely to arise. It is to these situations that this book will be addressed.

REFERENCES

1. MacKinnon, R and Michels, R: *The Psychiatric Interview.* WB Saunders, Philadelphia, 1971, Chapter 4.
2. Bibring, G: *Teaching medical psychology.* In Zinberg, NE (ED): *Psychiatry and Medical Practice in the General Hospital.* International Universities Press, New York, 1964.

3. JALOWIEC, A AND PWERS, M: *Stress and coping in hypertensive and emergency room patients.* Nurs Res 30:10, 1981.
4. LOEWENSTEIN, PL: *A Time to Love . . . A Time to Die.* Pyramid Books, New York, 1970.
5. MOWBRAY, A: *The Operation.* Signet Books, New York, 1972.

BIBLIOGRAPHY

COOK, S: *Second Life.* Simon & Schuster, New York, 1981.
LEAR, M: *Heartsounds.* Simon & Schuster, New York, 1980.
MEE, C, JR: *Seizure.* M Evans, New York, 1978.
POND, J: *Surviving.* Ace Books, New York, 1979.
ROLLINS, B: *First You Cry.* American Library, New York, 1976.
RYAN, K AND CORNELIUS, A: *Private Battle.* Simon & Schuster, 1979.

2
The Individual Becomes a Patient

Lisa Robinson, R.N., Ph.D., F.A.A.N., C.S.

The person facing admission to a hospital is beset by a number of problems both internal and environmental. His dilemma becomes more complex as he is transformed by the admission procedure from a person into a patient. Initially, he is given a name band to wear around his wrist. Henceforth his identity will be checked by a cursory glance at his arm rather than a vocal query. This communicates to the patient the lessened importance of his intellectual processes. Next, an institutional gown helps the sick person to exchange his role as a functioning adult for that of a patient. He is further guided into the ways of patientdom by being encouraged to go to bed. It is routine in the hospital to insist that a newly admitted patient get undressed and into bed even though the patient may be quite well, for example, a candidate for rhinoplasty. He is encouraged to slip into a hospital gown and retire to await the house officer's examination. Sometimes the examination does not take place for many hours.

Once in bed the individual is placed in the physical attitude of an infant on his back surrounded by caregiving people. In this vulnerable position, the sick person is expected to accept passively the scrutiny and prodding of his body by strangers. Questions of the most intimate nature are to be answered matter-of-factly. Specimens of various bodily products are to be dispensed upon request. These tasks involve the denial of such natural responses as fear, anger, and indignation. The sick adult has made a tacit agreement with the institution that he will proffer his body in exchange for intervention in his disease process. The intellectual and emotional components of that body are, at this point, denied expression.

The early hours of hospitalization provide an abundant set of cues to the patient that encourage his regression to earlier, less mature levels of behavior and response. The caregiving people tend to say little, since their presence has a task orientation. This communicates to the patient that conversation is of secondary importance. Owing partially to his illness and partially to the focus of the staff, the patient's bodily symptoms and needs become more important to him than anything else. It is noteworthy that patients rarely turn on their lights and request the nurse to stay with them because they are lonely or afraid. More likely patients will complain, when their lights are answered, that they have fleeting pains or need water or believe the bedpan might be necessary. Patients complain more of pain at night than during the daylight hours. This suggests, again, that it is really psychological support that is needed, rather than analgesics. The night is lonely, forbidding, and unfriendly. Patients rarely seek companionship and conversation; more often than not, the plea is for medicine or some type of physical manipulation. The patient learns that the use of body language is expedient.

Another lesson quickly learned during hospitalization is the importance of meals. They provide one of the few predictable diversions of the day. After a short period in the hospital, patients find themselves spending an inordinate amount of time choosing menus, anticipating meals, and evaluating their food. This preoccupation with food is reminiscent of earlier levels of development.

Still another trend toward regression is established by the hospital routine that requires the daily inquiry into colonic function. Is there any nurse on the evening shift who has not asked her patients if their bowels moved that day? This is doubtlessly a necessary part of the daily routine in order to make up the 8:00 P.M. cathartic list; however, it also serves to focus the patient's attention and anxieties upon his stool. Patients tend, eventually, to think a great deal about their alimentary tracts, from the mouth all the way through to the anus. This is so commonplace as to be considered an invariable part of the patient role.

Communications are altered in the hospital. The individual finds the usual mode of social intercourse inadequate in familiarizing him-

8

self with the new environment. Neither the hurried nurse nor the harried resident has the time to indulge in those social amenities that permit strangers to become acquainted. The patient finds much evidence to substantiate his preconscious awareness that his value to the institution lies in his performing the role of patient in a manner that is congruent with the system. The patient finds his personal identity suppressed as his institutional image emerges.

In a relatively short time, the patient is able to observe that the routine around him is established and implemented without his expressed wishes being considered. His assistance or cooperation is not really necessary for the ongoing operation. Meals, baths, medications, and treatments are administered in harmony with the schedule of the hospital. The patient is expected to submit to the system. Individuality threatens its efficiency.

Another facet of the patient role is that of the denial of sexuality. Male and female patients are attended by staff of both sexes. Types of physical contact considered inappropriate in a social setting become permissible in the hospital. The female nurse often has reason to touch the naked skin of her male patient. She administers injections of medication in the buttocks of many patients, male and female. She rubs their backs. She washes them. The male nurse, performing the same tasks as his female counterpart, administers to patients of both sexes. Such intimate contact would be considered inappropriate in a nonmedical relationship, but the nurse-patient contract condones such activity. Concomitant emotional reactions to these relationships are presumably not felt. In actuality, patients do respond to the touch of their caregivers, and their responses tend to merge with other feelings and behavior. Anxiety is engendered and is expressed in numerous ways. One major means of coping with anxiety is through regression. This defense is used by all patients to some extent. It is a helpful process that permits the patient to tolerate the psychological bombardment to which he is exposed and renders him capable of tolerating hospitalization.

The patient becomes markedly self-centered as his hospitalization progresses. Though he may intellectually recognize that he is only one of many patients, emotionally he needs to be certain that those caring for him are consistently interested in him and in his welfare. That he sees himself in possible jeopardy is related to his passive-dependent position. As has been previously described, food, medication, and treatments are administered within the hospital system by the nurse. The patient is neither expected nor encouraged to take an active part in procuring these daily necessities. He is considered a good patient if he passively accepts what is offered. The patient is physically and psychologically dependent upon the hospital and, more specifically, upon his nurse for his daily needs.

Besides the external pressures that cause the individual as a patient to conform to the system, there are internal issues that also promote this change. One of these internal issues is the alteration of body image during illness. The affected part of the body takes on special meaning. The ill person may regard it as something independent, something that needs special care. He may treat the injured or ill parts of himself as an anxious parent treats a sick child. Certain parts of the body have been invested with special meaning, and these areas, when injured or malfunctioning, will cause greater anxiety and promote more hovering attention. The skin, facial structures, head, genitals, and breasts represent highly valued parts of human anatomy. When these areas are involved in injury or illness, the patient's heightened apprehension may cause further regression. Mechanisms such as denial, repression, or compensation may help defend the patient from his anxiety.

Pain is another internal problem for the patient. The experience of pain causes isolation, since it is a very personal matter that cannot be readily shared by another. Because the patient can neither assess the pain objectively nor describe it qualitatively, he does not possess the means to share his experience with others. The discomfort itself is stressful. The patient's inability to communicate its character makes the pain more traumatizing. His efforts to control it are fruitless. The situation worsens. Thus pain, because of its many ramifications, is a very disorganizing experience. It promotes anxiety, which is itself experienced as additional pain. The sick person in the face of such a thoroughly overwhelming experience tends to cope, again, through regression.

Hospitalization itself has symbolic meaning. To some it means an affirmation of the inability to deal with the problems of everyday living; it is an admission that the illness is not merely a temporary indisposition. It may mean the confirmation of a fear of impending death. All these thoughts are more stressful because the patient is separated from friends and family.

The person—now patient—has been transformed from an autonomous, independently functioning, productive adult into a dependent, regressed, passive individual. This is not an indictment of the hospital but a descriptive analysis of the real and necessary process that takes Mr. John Doe away from his Sunday morning lawn mowing and changes him into the case of infectious hepatitis in Room 314. Without modifications in his mode of living and operating, Mr. Doe would be unable to tolerate hospitalization.

These factors in the external environment, coupled with the patient's internal life (that is, his fantasies and past experiences), influence the patient's behavior throughout his hospitalization.

If there is a unifying principle with which one might structure the psychological care of the individual who is becoming a patient, it is probably that the patient should be impressed with his likeness to those caring for him. Caregiving people should communicate to patients that they—the caregivers—have some awareness of the patient's feelings because, as fellow human beings, they have felt as their patients do—frightened, wary, lonely, sad, resigned. It is unnecessary and usually inappropriate to make these statements in a didactic manner; however, they can be communicated. The admitting staff member may sit in the patient's room and fill in the required papers as the patient gives information. She may comment on the suddenness of the patient's admission to the hospital and his attendant feelings. The nurse may venture a spoken thought such as, "It must be pretty upsetting to come into the hospital so suddenly," or, if the admission is an elective one, "It seems difficult for all of us to come into a place like the hospital. At least, *I've* felt uncomfortable. I'd like to try to make this easier for you, if I can."

If hospital staffing patterns permit, it is invaluable to assign a member of the nursing staff to each patient on a regular basis. In this way the patient can come to know one individual as a *real* person, not unlike himself. This helps the patient to assume his required role in the hospital without feeling divested of all that is himself as a human being. He need not resort to depersonalization in an effort to withstand the anonymity and the mechanization that the technological age has fostered in the hospital.

I recall vividly my own feelings after a lumbar puncture that had been anticipated with dread. A week's hospitalization preceded the procedure. Finally, the draped tray was brought in by an uninterested-looking aide. She said nothing, placed the tray on a table, and left.

The doctor arrived an hour later. One can imagine my thoughts, fantasies, and feelings during that hour. The procedure was accomplished with minor problems when a nerve was pierced. Small talk was attempted between patient and doctor during the proceedings. It seemed perversely amusing that while my *back* presented an impersonal vista to the doctor, my *front* was a mass of clenched muscles, with eyes shut tightly and hand clutched in that of the assisting nurse.

When the spinal fluid was obtained and measurements made, the needle was withdrawn, goodbyes were said, and the doctor left. The nurse stayed. She pulled a chair to the flattened bed and held my hand. I cried and cried, releasing all the pent-up feelings from a week of dreaded anticipation, from the helpless madness of having to submit to something that was painful, from the anger at the person who caused the pain. The nurse squeezed my hand and her eyes grew misty too. She said, "I'm so sorry. I know that hurt." It helped me to know that another human being—a friend—cared.

BIBLIOGRAPHY

GRAVELL, C: *The patient process: Understanding how a person has become a patient.* Nurs Times 77:144, 1981

JANIS, L: *Psychological Stress.* John Wiley & Sons, London, 1958.

LEDERER, H: *How the sick view their world.* In SKIPPER, J AND LEONARD, R (EDS): *Social Interaction and Patient Care.* JB Lippincott, Philadelphia, 1965.

NICKSIC, E: *Problem patients or problem nurses?* Nurs Outlook 29:317, 1981.

RICHARDS, C: *Communicating, communications—The patient's point of view.* Nurs 81, 7:1189, 1981.

STRAUSS, A, ET AL: *Patient's work in the technological hospital: Illness is more than passive suffering.* Nurs Outlook, 29:404, 1981.

3
The Patient Before Surgery

Lisa Robinson, R.N., Ph.D., F.A.A.N., C.S.

The patient who decides to undergo surgery has made an intellectual decision: He will submit to an operative procedure in order to correct some health problem. He has put aside his own opinion because he recognizes the superiority of his doctor's judgment. He has also repressed his own natural antipathy to bodily injury, unconsciousness, and lack of control.

He probably is not aware of these thoughts. Upon admission to the unit he feels some apprehension, perhaps some foreboding, but he accepts this as normal fear of new things—hospital, smells, people, and so forth. It is a rare patient who observes and verbalizes his ambivalence about surgery, yet it is operant. The patient behaves in a rational manner, recognizes the need for surgery, and agrees to submit. At an unconscious level, however, the patient must cope with his fears. This intrapsychic struggle causes conflict and anxiety. It is part of the apprehension that the patient experiences as he enters the hospital.

The nurse can be particularly supportive if she tells the patient what will be done to him during the hours prior to surgery. An explanation of blood tests and urinalysis is indicated. If the nurse knows whether a venipuncture or finger stick will be done, she should inform the patient. If an electrocardiogram is scheduled, the patient should be told about it. Sometimes the leads frighten a patient who thinks he will experience an electric shock. Therefore one should tell the patient that the procedure is painless and that he will feel nothing except the application of jelly and the attachment of the electrodes. If the patient is to undergo a major operation that will necessitate the extended use of recovery room or intensive care facilities, he should have the opportunity preoperatively to meet the nurses who will care for him.

The evening prior to surgery is particularly difficult for the patient. It is at this time that he must struggle with his misgivings and fears. Nighttime brings darkness, and the patient becomes aware that he is enclosed by hospital walls. The familiar surroundings outside are shrouded in darkness; the support of visitors and family is withdrawn and the patient is alone. The distant noises of the hospital punctuate the patient's loneliness and fear of the unknown. Rubber soles on linoleum, the flush of the hopper, and the sound of a hissing autoclave all remind the patient that he is in a strange and dangerous place.

As the time for sleep approaches, many patients begin to think of home, their families, separation, even death. Thoughts turn to pain and the experience of becoming anesthetized. It is no wonder that the aide coming into the patient's room to give evening care or the nurse bringing the sleeping pill finds a quiet, morose, or even tearful patient. It is not useful to explain that there is nothing to cry about. Actually, there is!

This is a time when human warmth and sensitivity are most requisite. The ability to tolerate crying and verbalizations of fear is necessary. To be helpful, the nurse needs to take the time to sit and listen to the patient. She cannot completely allay the patient's anxiety, because some of the patient's fears are not conscious. She can ask the patient directly about his major concerns and give him information that may be at variance with his fantasies. This transaction will in itself reduce anxiety. She can let the patient know that he has competent medical and nursing care. She can inform the patient that she will remain available to him. She can reassure him by saying that his fears are normal and that the sleeping pill will help him rest. She can help the patient to relax by giving him a back rub and listening quietly as he talks or by permitting the patient to remain silent.

On the day of surgery it is thoughtful to allow the patient to sleep as late as he can. Washing should be done when the patient feels like it. If possible, the patient should be permitted a tub bath or shower, since it will probably be the last for a while. Hospital gown and intravenous paraphernalia should be kept out of the room until it is time for their use. These things are frightening, and it is unkind to alarm the patient prematurely. Dentures, wedding band, and other removable objects should not be taken away until absolutely necessary. Wait until just prior to the arrival of the operating room stretcher, since removing them is traumatizing. Taking away possessions and one's mobility symbolically alters identity. Whatever the patient has brought into the hospital probably has special significance to him or the patient would have left these possessions at home, where they would be infinitely safer. Most persons feel denuded without their dentures; they cannot see clearly without glasses nor hear adequately without hearing aids. The loss of religious medals and wedding bands symbolically separates the patient from that which is intimate and reassuring. The patient is being asked to go into the feared unknown without protection. The IV and the hospital gown preclude any possibility of fantasied escape. Postponing these procedures helps the patient maintain his sense of intact identity for as long as possible. While an individual feels his old self, he can better cope with the stresses imposed by new experiences. The means of coping are closely bound up with an individual's sense of self.

It is difficult to imagine the feelings of the sedated, preoperative patient unless surgery has been experienced first hand. Giving up his watch, rings, glasses, or teeth also makes the patient overaware of his impending danger. It means that the hour of separation and unawareness is near. The hospital gown hardly covers the body. The patient feels naked and afraid.

The patients' fantasies are sometimes overwhelming as he allows himself to be placed on the stretcher and covered with a sheet. He is sedated and feels incapable of normal alertness. As the stretcher is withdrawn from the room and the familiar nurse disappears, the patient is afraid. He is nude, sedated, strapped down, and in the hands of an unfamiliar orderly. These fears, coupled with the patient's anxiety about the surgery, can give rise to overwhelming terror.

If at all possible, a familiar nurse or aide should accompany the patient to the operating suite. The sight of the ceiling gliding by, the coldness and hardness of the stretcher, and the sight of strange people's faces passing in the hall add to the patient's foreboding. If the patient wears glasses this experience is still worse, for they have been removed and he sees only blurs and shadows. The wait for the elevator is interminable. At this time, quiet conversation can be quite reinforcing. A hand casually laid on the patient's hand means so much. Since fear of the unknown and sedation are powerful causes of regression, the patient may be unable to experience *verbal* interaction as supportive, whereas nonverbal, physical transactions communicate concern and closeness. Preoperative medication and fear may cause tachycardia, a clammy feeling of the skin, and often nausea. The touch of a warm hand brings comfort.

Once they are in the operating room, there is little the nurse can do but stay close by and help the patient realize that the eyes behind the mask really belong to a feeling, concerned nurse. Soon anesthesia will crowd out the multitudinous fears and fantasies.

BIBLIOGRAPHY

ADAMSON, J, ET AL: *The psychic significance of parts of the body in surgery.* In HOWELL, J (ED): *Modern Perspectives in the Psychiatric Aspects of Surgery.* Brunner/Mazel, New York, 1976.

HAVEN, L, ET AL: *Reducing the patient's fear of the recovery room.* RN 38:28, 1974.

TITCHENER, J AND LEVINE, M: *Surgery as a Human Experience.* Oxford University Press, New York, 1960.

4
The Crying Patient

Lisa Robinson, R.N., Ph.D., F.A.A.N., C.S.

Crying is a form of communication. In the American culture it is tolerated in children but discouraged as verbal skills develop. The early years are accompanied by admonishments such as "Now dear, there is nothing to cry about," or "Act like a big boy now. You don't want the doctor to think you are a baby." Such parental pressures do not go unheeded. As the child grows into an adult, along with bladder and bowel controls and his awareness of other social amenities, he develops an unconsciously motivated prohibition concerning crying.

This prohibition is operant in the adult who fights for control of his crying or forbids himself to weep at all. This person usually does not connect his strict control with the admonishments of his childhood. When crying, he is aware of a feeling of discomfort ranging from the vaguest to the most severe level of anxiety. Some individuals experience tension with the awareness of any feeling. Men are less likely than women to relax this control. Tears are considered feminine, a sign of weakness, or a demonstration of inadequacy. It is significant that the incidence of ulcers is greater in men than in women. Though it is not proven, one can hypothesize that the male, being unable to express his tension through rather harmless crying, is forced to endure stressful feelings until they are expressed through traumatized tissue. Women seem more able than men to allow themselves to weep occasionally.

Crying conveys discouragement, sadness, pain, frustration, or anger. Sometimes it is a plea for help. The tearful patient who is seeking help through his tears may not know why he is crying or why he wishes aid. When asked "Why are you crying?" or "What is the matter?" the patient may be unable to give a reasonable explanation. He may then feel that because he does not have a ready answer his tears are not justified and that he must be quiet. It is for this reason that one must ask for explanations only after some forethought.

Though the patient may not have a conscious explanation for his crying, there is a reason for it. Crying is communication. It is an expression of some feeling. If the patient senses that the nurse cannot tolerate his tears, he feels that she cannot accept his feelings. Thus it is wise to allow the patient to cry. When the episode is over, exploration of its cause or causes can be initiated.

All too often when a nurse walks into a patient's room and finds him crying, she feels anxious. She wonders what is happening to the patient. The patient realizes only that he is experiencing discomfort. The nurse feels constrained and compelled to stop her patient's tears. She tries a variety of means to stop him, without finding out what this indirect communication means. The message is shut off with "Don't worry, dear. You have nothing to be afraid of. You are going to be all right," or "There now, you have a wonderful doctor."

It is very important to decode the patient's message. In order to do that, however, the nurse must be able to tolerate her own feelings of discomfort in the presence of the crying patient. It is important for the patient to see that his crying can be tolerated. This implies that his feelings are acceptable. It is possible that the real reason for the tears will never be realized consciously; however, the nurse's acceptance of the general situation is supportive.

The nurse sometimes feels that she must do *something*. This something turns out to be stopping the patient's tears. Basically, this is attempting to control the patient. It is useful for the nurse to realize that she can control only one human being—herself. If she is aware of her own feelings of discomfort and can function in spite of them, she will be less prone to attempt control of the patient.

When confronted with crying, the nurse will find it useful to focus on the patient's feelings. Such comments as "You must be very unhappy," or "You seem so uncomfortable," permit the patient to explore his reasons for crying. The nurse has not implied that the patient must stop weeping. Another introductory statement that does not assign a meaning to the crying is, "I'd like to help you. Can you tell me about your thoughts and feelings right now?"

Occasionally a person cries simply to release tension. Physical contact is comforting at these times. A hand on the patient's shoulder or arm or a box of tissues placed conveniently near—these are signs of warm, human caring.

The following cases demonstrate two entirely different meanings expressed in the same type of behavior.

Mrs. McS., a 56-year-old housewife, was admitted to the hospital because of an orthopedic problem. The patient was a large-boned, rather unattractive woman. She was referred to the clinical specialist by the staff nurses, who reported that Mrs. McS. cried all day and needed someone to talk to.

When seen by the interviewer, Mrs. McS. described the inadequate nursing care she had received. This part of her conversation was brief. Her description of home and family was far more lengthy and shed light on her crying problem in the hospital. It developed that this patient was the primary support of a family of six that included the patient, a semiretired husband, a senile father, a 36-year-old, severely mentally retarded son, a 74-year-old mother, and a 7-year-old granddaughter. The patient kept house for this heterogeneous group. She tried to make ends meet with retirement and Social Security checks. The retarded son posed a chronic problem that she recognized as insoluble. Institutionalization would eventually be necessary, but the patient wanted to keep her child at home as long as possible. The father was destined for a state institution. Mrs. McS. was the only strong one in this group and all problems were heaped on her shoulders. She bore these tribulations with equanimity.

When she was admitted to the orthopedic service, Mrs. McS. was placed in traction. She required assistance with her most basic needs. For a woman who had been unusually self-sufficient this was a difficult adjustment to make. Also, her family visited her daily and continued to deluge her with problems she could not possibly handle from her sickbed. When she was not preoccupied with thoughts of her foundering family, she was bothered by chronic pain. When she needed help, she had to wait until someone came to the bedside.

Eventually the pain, the frustration, and the hopelessness of her chronic problems overwhelmed her and Mrs. McS. could only cry. Words could not possibly express her feelings. There were few measures that the nurse could take to make Mrs. McS. more comfortable. This was a situation in which sitting, listening, and sharing the moment was all that could be offered.

Mr. W. was a 45-year-old salesman who was admitted to the intensive care unit following a myocardial infarction. The nurses observed that this patient always joked with them. He gave no indication that he was worried or uncomfortable.

Whenever his wife visited, Mr. W.'s demeanor reversed itself. He became tearful and depressed. Mrs. W. told the nurses that she was concerned because Mr. W. seemed so depressed. He clung to her and cried during their entire visit each time.

The nurses called the interviewer. She did not talk directly to the patient because of the nature of his relationship with the nurses but talked with Mrs. W. instead. Mrs. W. described her husband as being terrified of his illness. He said little to her, but when he did talk his thoughts were obviously about separation and death. He believed that he would not leave the hospital alive. His crying was apparently an expression of his true feelings. Mr. W. was depressed and terror-stricken.

The nurses were encouraged to ignore Mr. W.'s joking and levity. They were to approach him in a friendly way but not to permit themselves to become involved in Mr. W.'s denial of his feelings. They were asked to spend additional time with him when possible, in order that Mr. W. might ventilate some of his thoughts and feelings.

This regimen was useful. Soon Mrs. W. noticed that her husband seemed less tearful during her visits. His conversations did not center on death. Mr. W. was apparently able to share some of his thoughts with those caring for him. As often happens with patients who are afraid, voicing his thoughts helped to alter the anxiety-provoking component in them.

It has been said and is believed by many caregiving workers that specific behaviors need not indicate specific disorders. The behaviors have a meaning that is peculiar to the individual, and that individual—and thus the meaning of his behavior—is unique. We have looked at several possible meanings implicit in crying: futility, frustration, hopelessness, depression, and fear.

For a small group of patients, either chronically and severely emotionally handicapped or grossly regressed on an acute basis secondary to hospitalization, crying may represent the only available means of communication. As mentioned, this group of patients is small, and the nurse will rarely encounter such a problem. However, when she does, she will base her diagnosis on the following criteria: (1) The patient cries in the presence of the majority of the staff. (2) He does not appear able to translate his communication into verbal terms. (3) Staff have tried individually and as a group to understand the patient's meaning and have been unable to discover a clue which might alter the interpersonal situation. The nurse's conclusion will be that the crying does not have one meaning at all but has multiple meanings.

Staff can accept the situation as an unchangeable one, that is, they can accept their inability to understand the patient. They will, of necessity, work in the dark with that patient, because there is no relatedness where there is no understanding. Such is often the case when one nurses the patient with acute brain trauma or the patient is decerebrate. On the other hand, staff may believe that change is possible, that fuller communication and understanding can take place vis à vis the patient. Criteria upon which to base such a decision are the patient's state of consciousness, his apparent awareness of staff's presence, and any degree of modification in his behavior in the presence of one staff member as compared with another or with visitors.

For those patients in whom change seems possible, staff must decide the direction of change and the means of shaping or modifying the behavior. This is a difficult concept to work with because it contradicts the notion that all behavior has meaning and (implicit in that idea) that each patient has a right to his own particular means of expression. Nonetheless, in the small percentage of patients described, *no* understanding is occurring and, right or wrong, a group of people desire to help the patient to learn a more effective means of relating. When the ethical factor is resolved, staff can outline an approach to the problem. If the patient cries with all staff members at all times, staff should decide on a basic pattern for their own behavior as they encounter the patient. It is useful to ask the patient what it is that he is trying to say. If he does not answer or if the answer is not understandable, the patient should be told that the nurse does not understand. She should be sure that the patient knows the nurse sincerely wishes to help but is unable to without further information. If the patient *does* respond in a meaningful way then the nurse can react accordingly. If the patient continues to respond in a way that cannot be understood, the nurse *must* maintain her position, letting the patient know that she wants to help but does not know how without the patient's direction. If the patient is actually capable of a better response and *if* the nurse can cope with her own anxiety sufficiently well that she does *not* initiate a hunt and peck operation in order to *guess* the patient's needs, the patient is likely to reach for a more effective means of communication. When this happens, the nurse should respond as quickly as possible so that there is a bond established in the patient's mind between his behavior and the nurse's response. This will reinforce the behavior.

A case in point is R.C., a 37-year-old stripper, who was admitted to the hospital via the emergency room. She complained of severe abdominal pain which was beginning to localize in the lower right quadrant. It was decided that the patient had appendicitis, and she was sent to surgery. The patient was placed on service because she did not have adequate financial resources for private care.

The recovery room notes showed that R.C. reacted quickly postoperatively, and she was transferred to the ward. There she was oriented to the unit, and staff tried to get to her sometime during their shift to introduce themselves. The patient complained several times of discomfort for which she was medicated. The nurses' notes of the following day were the first to portend trouble. R.C. cried intermittently all day. Staff were solicitous but unable to understand the basic problem. The third day was a repetition of the second. Staff believed that the patient might be having difficulties with flatulence. They encouraged ambulation. Still the patient moaned and wept quietly. Finally the staff, feeling ineffective and anxious about R.C., held a conference. They decided to try to modify the patient's means of communication.

The fourth day brought some change in the patient in the form of monosyllabic demands. During the three shifts that day, staff were aware of a feeling that they had in the presence of the patient which they could characterize only as oddly negative. The fifth day was like the fourth in that the crying decreased even more, but as that behavior decreased, a definite hostile attitude toward the nurses increased. Staff were able to accept R.C.'s behavior, though they wondered about its origin. On the sixth day, one of the older LPNs decided to simply ask the patient what was wrong. She was ill prepared for the avalanche of words and feelings that poured from the patient as she described her bitterness about the surgery and the scar that would now end her means of livelihood. R.C. also verbalized her pent-up rage at the younger female personnel whom she said were better looking than she and did not have to "kill themselves making a buck" as R.C. did. The nurse brought this information to the change of shift report. It was decided to communicate with the resident who informed the group that a very low, small incision had been made on the patient because of her occupation. On rounds the next day, the patient was so informed, and she noted this herself when the sutures were removed. Staff noted an immediate change in R.C.'s attitude. She brightened noticeably.

After the patient's discharge, staff agreed that R.C.'s moaning and weeping probably represented, in the main, a combination of her anger at what appeared to be the enforced end of a career, plus her envy of other females around her whom she perceived to be more attractive than herself. By not accepting R.C.'s original response, staff helped her to mobilize her anger and to be able to ventilate it. Staff agreed that their special interest and effort with R.C. had been of value.

The following case illustrates the clinical management of a patient who cried continuously, not as a communication, but as a reflection of brain insult and emergent primitive behavior.

Dan, a 24-year-old single male, was brought to the emergency room by three friends. He had taken an undetermined amount of methadone earlier in the day. Later, his friends reported, he got into his car and backed it up with the driver's side door open. He hit a telephone pole and fell out of the car. His friends rushed to him and asked if he was all right. He denied injury, climbed back into the car, and drove to his apartment. The friends went off to class. When they returned to the apartment, they found Dan unconscious on the bed. He was barely breathing and blood seeped from his ears. The friends took him to the hospital.

While in the emergency room, Dan had a cardiac arrest and was resuscitated. He was then transferred to the intensive care unit. Upon admission, he experienced another cardiac arrest and was once more resuscitated. His blood pressure had to be maintained on Isuprel for the next three days. During that time he was noted to have no breath sounds on the left side, and a chest tube was inserted. At no time during the first seven days of hospitalization did the patient react to anything but deep, painful stimuli.

In the second week, Dan began to regain consciousness. He now convulsed when stimulated. During this time, a weakness on the right side was noted and an arteriogram was done. The results were negative. Dan's level of consciousness steadily improved. At the end of the second week, he was discharged from the intensive care unit to the regular patient unit. Staff observed him to be whiny, demanding, and uncooperative. He tried to smoke constantly and often dropped his lit cigarette butts on the sheets. When admonished about this he cried. Because of the weakness of his right side, he was given physical therapy. When the therapy was delayed or cancelled, as it was on a religious holiday, Dan sat in the hall and cried. Staff always asked Dan if they could help, and what was the nature of his distress, but the patient usually could not say. He simply wept louder and longer.

Eventually the nursing staff became quite uncomfortable and anxious about their patient's behavior because they could not alter his discomfort. The liaison nurse was called. She observed that Dan did not seem to be alert yet. She theorized that he was still cloudy from his head injury and that his whiny, crying behavior reflected postconcussion syndrome. She related to the staff that Dan probably reacted diffusely to incoming stimuli and that he would be more comfortable if the stimuli could be decreased. She also recommended a structuring of Dan's time, with some options open to him so that he could still feel an appropriate amount of autonomy. The nursing care plan was effective and Dan's behavior was observed to change.

BIBLIOGRAPHY

SMOYAK, S: *Is life the pits?* Imprint 28:34, 1981.

TOWNS, J: *How to communicate with a person in sorrow.* Nurs Forum, 19:300, 1980.

5

The Frightened Patient

Lisa Robinson, R.N., Ph.D., F.A.A.N., C.S.

Another culturally determined response is the adult's reaction to fright. Adults are uncomfortable verbalizing fear. They are likely to convert their feelings into somatic symptoms, to deny them, to hide them from others, or to escalate angry feelings to overcome the frightened ones.

People who are frightened experience a physiological response. They may perspire freely, feel a temperature change in the skin, or be aware of a sinking sensation in the stomach. In an extremely frightening situation, bladder control may be lost.

Some patients who are afraid do not display their fear openly. Men are more likely than women to have problems in this area, since in American culture the female is permitted overt expression of fright. Individuals who do not express their fear may develop physical symptoms that accomplish the objective of removing the individual from the threatening situation. Such is the case when a student facing a final examination develops such an excruciating headache that the test must be postponed. It should be kept in mind, however, that physiological response to fear does not always have symbolic meaning but can be the direct response to a real threat.

Denial of fright involves defensive operations that are unconscious. These defenses permit the individual to negate his fear. The person using denial does not recognize the real character of his discomfort. If an observer tells this person that he looks frightened, the individual is apt to reply that he is not. When denial is not effective, the individual may still consciously attempt to disguise his thoughts in the presence of others. In American culture verbalizing fear, like crying, is not common beyond childhood.

We see the anlages of this inhibition when a mother is overheard chiding her offspring for being afraid. Perhaps a nurse tells a pediatric patient, "Be a brave boy now," or a parent says, "Now, now, there is nothing to be afraid of." The child realizes that fear itself and the expression of fear are not acceptable.

When the child grows to adulthood, he no longer recalls his parents' admonishments, but the vestiges of this early training are present in his adult reaction to a fear-provoking experience. He may, as a patient facing a frightening situation, desire support from the nurse, but he cannot indicate this to her. Nurses who are perceptive about their patients' feelings tend to respond in a reassuring manner even though the need is not openly admitted or verbalized.

There are some patients who are so threatened by illness that they cannot permit themselves to become aware of their feelings. Such a realization would threaten their sense of identity. Such persons have learned in their formative years to deny the existence of their feelings, and thus they literally do not know *how* to feel. Their personalities have become structured in such a way that they have no means for confronting their feelings. To perceive feeling would be tantamount to destroying or significantly altering their sense of identity. These are the patients who behave hypercritically or become unusually demanding. They may seem obnoxious because of their aggressive, brazen behavior. These behavior patterns enable the patient to feel less afraid. The behavior should not be construed as a response to an environmental situation; it is actually an expression of the patient's inner turmoil. Such patients as these cannot accept support and succor from their caregivers, since accepting these attentions would necessitate a recognition of the fear.

This can be a complex nursing problem with a patient who has unmet dependency needs but has repressed them. The passive position into which he is forced as a patient who must be cared for can be extremely dangerous psychologically. Such a person will be gratified by passively receiving care, but a recognition of such feelings in himself can undermine his entire personality structure. Thus this patient will not cooperate with the treatment regimen. In this way, he circumvents the possibility of recognizing his needs or having these needs satisfied.

The following case demonstrates this type of problem. Mr. F., a 48-year-old taxi driver, was brought into the emergency room after suffering a myocardial infarction. According to his history, he had suffered his first heart attack 10 years previously. He had convalesced uneventfully after that episode and had gone home while continuing with anticoagulants. He was now admitted to the intensive care unit. The nurses found Mr. F. to be very uncooperative. He refused to stay in bed, got up to go to the bathroom, fed himself, and smoked. Occasionally, while being bathed, Mr. F. would expose himself and ask the nurse if she was embarrassed. His conversation centered on speculation as to his ability to achieve orgasm. The nurses caring for this patient were uncomfortable and sought consultation. They knew that Mr. F. was terribly frightened and was aware that he might be facing possible death. The nurses formed a plan to tell him without undue emotion that they were uncomfortable when he exposed himself. They admitted their discomfort and asked him to behave more appropriately in their presence. This strategy accomplished several things. First, it demonstrated to the patient that the nurses were aware of him because of their responding to him. Second, the nurses admitted their discomfort, which seemed to be, at least superficially, a goal of the patient. Third, the nurses, through their comments, indicated an awareness of Mr. F.'s masculinity, that is to say, they reacted to his sexual behavior. Last, their request gave the patient some external controls.

Mr. F. was able to comply. Later in the hospitalization, the nurses attempted to explore with him the reasons for his behavior. They introduced the topic by saying, "You must have been very frightened to act as you did." Mr. F. was not able to admit his fears, but he did become more cooperative. He never was able to follow the treatment regimen completely but managed to maintain his equilibrium with only an occasional stolen cigarette or a short hike up the hall. He was finally discharged as improved. The nurses later heard that he was brought back to the emergency room dead on arrival after attempting coitus. They could only speculate that his identification was so tenuous that Mr. F. had had to deny his illness at the cost of his life.

It is not uncommon to observe sexually oriented behavior in patients who are overwhelmed by fear. The basis of this behavior is that the anxiety experienced by the patient is so great that he regresses. His sexual behavior is not an expression of adult sexuality but rather a reflection of narcissism and pregenital strivings. (The underlying anxiety might have been expressed in other areas besides the sexual.)

Male patients who are forced into positions of dependency and passive acceptance, such as those who are ordered to be on complete bed rest because of a myocardial infarction, frequently find this situation untenable. They feel the threatened loss of self-image. Indeed, they are aware of the possibility of loss of life itself. In an effort to buffer themselves against these overwhelming realizations, the existence of illness is denied. Panic is combated by focusing on the penis—that which is indisputably male, a symbol of procreativity. Mr. F. may unconsciously have been requesting assurance from the nurses that he was still a man, that is to say, that his illness and hospitalization had not deprived him of his maleness, his identity.

Sexually oriented behavior is also a means of denying the severity of the illness. It says, in effect, *I am not desperately ill. I can and will pursue my normal sexual inclinations.* The patient is indirectly showing his resolution to behave as if he were enjoying a normal state of health.

Sexuality is frequently confused with the need for intimacy by both the sick and well. All people have a need to be close to and understood by others. When under the stress of severe illness, patients sometimes act as if they are seeking sexual union when actually their need is for closeness, reassurance that they will not die, and understanding of their fears. Also some people who need closeness are afraid of it, and they too sexualize the need in order to defend against the intimacy that they fear.

Another explanation of sexual behavior, when it is aggressive in nature, concerns the patient's inability to tolerate the recognition of his dependency needs. To some people who have unresolved conflict in this area, the recognition of longings for dependency would de-

stroy their defensive use of the mechanism of co
individuals, the realization that they are not con
and strong would mean loss of identity. For the
gression can be a means of reacting against the r
dependent. By acting aggressively, the patie
longing. Gratification of his dependency need
because the nurse who might respond positively is frightened and
withdraws.

Still another facet of this type of behavior is its defensive nature in
the personality with strong latent homosexual strivings. A segment of
the population is able to relate heterosexually only at a great expendi-
ture of energy directed toward the suppression of homosexual needs.
The nursing care received by such a patient can stimulate these latter
feelings, causing the patient great discomfort, even threatening the
individual's psychic integration. In order to compensate, the patient
may behave in a hypermasculine manner in order to feel less threatened.

One of the underlying theories in the management of the frightened patient is to decrease the fright by increasing the patient's control. Though not satisfactorily investigated as yet, it appears that the
individual who feels greater control also feels that he can predict outcomes and prepare for them so that he is essentially less vulnerable.

A child once told me how terrified she felt when wrapped in a
blanket so that she was effectively restrained for blood samples to be
drawn. One day, in the clinic, the physician sat the child up on the
examining table, matter of factly told her about the need for a venipuncture, and then collected the specimen. The child compared the
approaches and concluded that: "It didn't hurt when (the doctor) let
me sit up." From the child's report, it might be concluded that her
physical position permitted her greater control. Lying supine and im-
mobilized offered no opportunity for response; sitting up, she had
sufficient *potential* for protecting herself—that is, for control—that she
did not *need* to react with fear or panic.

A different type of situation is seen in the case of Mr. D., a 54-year-
old diabetic who was admitted to the surgical service because of an
infected ankle that was not healing well. The ankle continued to
worsen in spite of a stringent medical regimen. Finally, the surgeons

ed to consult and a below-the-knee amputation was decided
The patient was informed, and he seemed, when signing the
rative permit, to understand. When Mr. D. returned from surgery, he complained of intense pain that did not subside for three
days. The patient was medicated as often as possible for his discomfort. Mr. D. was most uncooperative in keeping the stump elevated.
He was restless, possibly as a result of pain, and the leg was more
often under the pillow than on top of it. On the fourth day, the ban-
dages showed large quantities of bright red blood. The patient was
hemorrhaging badly and had to be returned to the operating room
where the stump was revised. Postoperatively, Mr. D. again complained. He did not, however, move his limb from its elevated position. The nurses were concerned about this patient. They felt that his
pain must be related to anxiety, and they theorized that moving his
stump after the first operation might have represented an attempt to
gain greater self-control. If this was the case, the psychological picture
was even bleaker after the second surgery, for the fear and anxiety
remained, but the patient did not demonstrate any means of coping
with it.

A conference was scheduled. Fear, anxiety, and the meaning of
loss of a body part were discussed—the latter in terms of its equiva-
lence to loss of a loved one.[1] The grieving process was compared with
this patient's behavior. Out of the discussion came a plan to recognize
Mr. D.'s *need* to grieve for his lost limb. Staff agreed to create an environment in which he could be sad and introspective. They agreed to
try to control their own impulses to say, "It's all right, Mr. D. Everything is fine now." Next the staff turned their attention to decreasing
the patient's fear and anxiety. They identified situations in which Mr.
D. could have increased control of his environment. The group mentioned choice of time for morning care, selection of menus, and planning of day's activities as means of giving the patient control. They
also discussed going to the patient when possible and *asking* if they
might sit and visit. The group noted that each person had to be prepared to leave if Mr. D. did not wish company and to not react defen-
sively to the possible rejection.

The plan was effective. It was noted in the next seven days that Mr.
D. changed. His need for pain medication decreased, he became

more verbal, and he seemed brighter. Staff felt comfortable in planning with Physical Medicine for the patient's course of rehabilitation and discharge.

It is important to remember that these formulations are only useful constructs. They are not validated truths but attempts to explain normal and aberrant behavior. As such, these and other dynamic formulations must be looked upon as guidelines. When one is working out nursing care plans, constructs such as those described can be useful in attempting to explain patient behavior and in structuring means to meet patients' needs.

REFERENCES

1. ROSEN, V: *The role of denial in acute postoperative affective reactions following removal of body parts.* Psychosom Med 12:354, 1954.

BIBLIOGRAPHY

KNOWLES, R: *Dealing with feelings: Managing anxiety Part I.* Am J Nurs 81:110, 1981.

CASSEM, N AND HACKETT, T: *The setting of intensive care.* In HACKETT, T AND CASSEM, N (EDS): *Massachusetts General Hospital Handbook of General Hospital Psychiatry.* CV Mosby, St. Louis, 1978.

LYNCH, J: *The Broken Heart: The Medical Consequences of Loneliness.* Basic Books, New York, 1977.

PRITCHARD, P: *Stress and anxiety in physical illness: The role of the general nurse.* Nurs Times 77:162, 1981.

6
The Disoriented Patient

Lisa Robinson, R.N., Ph.D., F.A.A.N., C.S.

The disoriented patient poses a severe nursing problem in the general hospital setting. Though this kind of problem is accepted and treated with relative facility in the psychiatric setting, it is not dealt with as easily in the daily management of patients hospitalized for acute medical problems.

Disorientation is most often observed in senile and senescent patients. The problem of increased disorientation as night draws near, with remission of the symptoms by dawn, is so common among elderly hospitalized patients that it has earned the name sundowner's disease.

Symptoms ranging from confusion to gross disorientation can also be observed in patients who have had high temperatures or in patients recovering from anesthesia or seizures. If one looks closely, some degree of disorientation can be observed in almost all patients who have survived critical surgery or illness. One needs only to visit the recovery room to observe patients who have undergone open heart surgery or the intensive care unit where victims of myocardial infarctions are convalescing in order to observe patients demonstrating a marked degree of disorientation.

The symptoms of disorientation are a vagueness about the identification of time, place, and person. This type of problem is always observed in patients who suffer from acute or chronic organic brain syndrome. At this stage and intensity of illness, the patient will appear drowsy and may doze most of the time. He will have a decreased attention span. Most important from the point of view of nursing intervention is the fact that the patient suffers from impaired perception and interpretation of external stimuli. He is likely to have impaired recent memory and retention. The patient is disoriented and regressed and may appear suspicious, depressed, or hostile. Acting out of sexual impulse is not uncommon. The patient in this condition is frightened. He may be assaultive, destructive, or suicidal.

Disorientation and delirium differ from postoperative psychosis. Disorientation is usually short-lived. Generally it is associated with high temperature, drug withdrawal, accumulation of metabolic products, or acute head injury. Delirium is a disturbance of reality testing on the perceptual level. It is accompanied by agitation and anxiety. If delusions or hallucinations occur, they are usually unstructured and lack the regressive quality of fixed psychotic thinking.

In postoperative psychosis, the disorder is predominantly in the patient's thinking. The restless quality of the delirious patient is not seen. Anxiety is not overtly demonstrated. The patient is delusional because his problem is at the conceptual and symbolic level of reality testing. Perceptual disturbances and disorientation are relatively rare. Psychotic symptoms appear without abnormal physiological conditions, and the duration is apt to be less predictable than in the case of delirium.

The patient who is disoriented or delirious needs to be reassured and reoriented. His ability to test reality needs to be strengthened and supported. The patient who becomes psychotic postoperatively must have more intensive care that focuses upon the elevation of the patient's feelings about himself. The psychotic patient's self-evaluations tend to involve feelings of worthlessness and dejection.

It is often very difficult to distinguish between delirium, disorientation, and postoperative psychosis. For this reason consultation for evaluation purposes may be sought with neurologists or psychiatrists. If these consultations determine that the patient is experiencing postoperative psychosis, antipsychotic medication may also be instituted to alter the patient's mental state.

Mr. S., a 53-year-old salesman, was admitted because of pain in the rectal area following bowel movements. He was diagnosed as having hemorrhoids, which were surgically removed. Postoperatively, Mr. S.

had a low-grade fever. He was unable to sleep at night and roamed the hall. The nurses noted Mr. S.'s confusion. His eyes seemed glazed, he cried frequently, and he refused medication. About four days after his operation, Mr. S. was found singing loudly. When his wife came to visit, he cautioned her to sit across the room from him, because there was ether around the bed.

A psychiatrist saw Mr. S. and prescribed Thorazine. The patient's disturbance was quickly controlled with the medication and nursing measures such as repeated identification of time, place, and person. A clock was put in the room, a wall calendar was displayed, and the daily newspaper was made available. The nursing staff did not argue with Mr. S. about his delusions but made it clear that their perceptions of the facts were different from his. With this regimen, the problem subsided quickly and Mr. S. made a good recovery.

Sometimes psychosis and senility meet in the same patient. Such a situation arose when Miss V. was admitted to the general hospital from a state mental institution. She was 77 years old and had been hospitalized for 30 years because of chronic schizophrenia. Miss V. was brought to the general hospital because she was bleeding rectally. It was thought that she had an operable lesion of the sigmoid.

Prior to surgery Miss V. presented no problems. She was placed on an open ward where constant surveillance was possible. The patient did not socialize but did occupy herself by sitting and rocking or pacing the floor, humming softly to herself. She ate well and was willing to attend to her own hygienic needs. After thorough work-up, the patient was ready for surgery. The doctors tried to tell Miss V. about the impending operation but she seemed unable to comprehend its nature.

When she was returned from the operating room, the operative note indicated that an abdominal perineal resection had been done. The staff waited and wondered. By the third postoperative day Miss V. was entirely conscious and alert. She pulled constantly at her naso-gastric tube, intravenous catheters, Foley, and Hemovacs. Mechanical restraint was the only means of insuring the continued placement of these necessities. The nurses spent as much time as they could at the bedside talking to the patient or simply touching her and letting her know that they were concerned. Eventually, Miss V. did manage to pull out her nasogastric tube and intravenous catheter. Both were left out since her condition seemed to warrant it. It was at this time that a diet was begun and the patient was approached about the care of her colostomy bag. What a fiasco! Miss V. seemed as intent on removing it as the nurse was intent on applying it. When the patient was not busy taking off her bag, she was picking at the bedding or at her few remaining tubes. The nursing staff was frustrated. They simply could not control Miss V.'s busy fingers.

During a team conference one of the aides suddenly brightened. She had an idea. Her little son (3 years old) had been given a thick string with large, colored, wooden beads. In the past two years he had enjoyed stringing them and wearing the necklaces he made, but now he had outgrown them. Why not string the beads, knot the string in order to prevent Miss V. from taking them off, and give the necklace to her to occupy her hands? The staff was interested in the outcome and waited patiently until the aide remembered to bring them. The necklace was presented to Miss V., who held them up, seemed to study them carefully, and fingered each one. From that day on, Miss V. was never seen without her beads. She even slept with them under her pillow. During the night, the nurse would occasionally hear a click, click, click as Miss V. awakened and fingered her beads in the dark. The remaining tubes and colostomy bag no longer presented a problem. They were ignored by the patient as she watched staff members and slid her beads along the string. When the patient was readied for discharge back to the state hospital, someone attempted to take the beads, but Miss V. would not give them up. Staff were happy to send them home with her, and they hoped that the beads would be a reminder to this older psychotic patient that people had been concerned and had cared for her.

At times, patients are admitted with very severe illnesses and a concurrent *acute* psychosis. It may be noted that the psychosis is abruptly terminated during the physical illness. This seems to occur so that all of the person's energy, including psychic energy, is available to focus on the life-threatening crisis.

Adult patients who are disoriented or delirious sometimes respond combatively. When this happens, the nurse should realize that her patient is in dire psychological distress. He may be delusional, as often occurs in postoperative psychosis, or he may be misinterpreting his environment because he is delirious. He may be striking out at an alien environment, as is seen in the case of the elderly disoriented patient. In any of these cases, the patient's perception of the world around him is as real to him as the nurse's perception of it is to her.

At times patients are combative because they are frightened. They do not regard verbal communication as an adequate means of expressing themselves. Such is the case when the patient is overwhelmed by stress and unable to use his defenses adequately. Fear and fantasies about fear-provoking objects can cause overwhelming stress. Illness itself or illness combined with sedating medication can render the patient unable to cope with stress. Drugs such as the phenothiazines and barbitals frequently sedate the patient to the point where he feels out of control and alarmed at his inability to respond appropriately. At this point, he lashes out combatively. One can attempt to understand this feeling of desperation in the following case.

Mrs. O., a 54-year-old married housewife, was admitted through the emergency room. Her record indicated a diagnosis of possible pancreatitis and malnutrition. The nurses discovered from the history that Mrs. O. had been a patient of the attending physician for many years. She was chronically ill as the result of heavy drinking. Mrs. O. presented no nursing problems for several days after admission. She looked quite ill and remained in bed. Her treatment regimen consisted of a high protein-high carbohydrate diet, vitamins, and nighttime sedation.

On the fourth day of hospitalization, Mrs. O. became irritable and demonstrated increasing agitation. The nurses were alarmed and requested consultation with me, the clinical specialist in psychiatry. Mrs. O. was in her bed in a private room. She looked quite ill. Her color was ashen, her hair and gown disheveled. The woman appeared to be grossly underweight. She was only moderately verbal, stopping often in the midst of a belabored verbal production to stare off into space.

The staff nurses and I later discussed Mrs. O. It was felt that the patient was going into delirium tremens. Her history of heavy drinking, the interval of time from admission to the onset of symptoms, plus the nature of her symptoms led the staff to feel assured of their diagnosis. It was decided that little could be done to stave off the clinical problem; however, the nurses could notify the doctor and watch the patient closely in order to be prepared to support and protect her.

Several hours later, I was requested to come immediately to the unit because Mrs. O. had become combative and unmanageable. The patient was found crouched in a corner of her room. She looked terrified. I said, "I am the nurse who visited you earlier, Mrs. O. Can I help you?" The patient did not respond. She did not indicate that she had heard. "You look very frightened, Mrs. O. Let me stay with you."

Still she did not answer. While I remained with the patient, immediate consultation was sought with the house officer. He ordered intramuscular paraldehyde. When the nurse entered the room with the medication, Mrs. O. crouched further down in the corner. Her mouth was curled into a snarl. The nurse said, "I want you to get into bed, Mrs. O. I have some medicine for you."

The patient made no move to comply. The nurse alternately tried cajoling and threatening. Not having intervened up to that point, I now said, "Mrs. O., the doctor is very anxious for you to have this medicine. He thinks it will help you to feel better."

"No. I won't take it," screamed Mrs. O.

"If you will not cooperate, we shall have to give it to you anyway," I said.

The patient sobbed and repeated that she would not allow the medication to be given. The nurse was then instructed to get enough help to lift Mrs. O. bodily. She returned with an orderly and two nurses. The patient saw the entourage and got into bed without further encouragement. The medication was administered. The group left the room, leaving one nurse to care for Mrs. O. Reinforced screening was placed in the window to prevent injury from a fall. The blinds were lowered. Mrs. O. slept much of the next 48 hours. A nurse was in constant attendance. The patient made an uneventful recovery from her delirium.

Nursing intervention for the care of this frightened, combative patient consisted, first, of notifying the patient that her discomfort was recognized. Second, the patient knew that a nurse wanted to remain with her. Had the patient been more verbal, the cause of her terror might have been explored. Third, the patient was told that she would be helped. When she resisted treatment, the patient was shown immediately that the staff could set limits and control her behavior when she was unable to do so herself. Such a demonstration, while it sounds cruel and brutal, is actually very reassuring. The patient sensed her inability to control her behavior, and this awareness created anxiety. External controls were comforting until she could assume responsibility for her own behavior.

When one is confronted with an uncooperative or combative patient such as Mrs. O. or a frightened patient, it is well not to cajole or threaten. Such maneuvers only cause further stress to the patient. It is far more humane to state matter of factly what must be done and to do it immediately. If mechanical restraints can be avoided, they should not be used. In the case of a patient who is delirious, restraints are particularly contraindicated. The patient is rendered incapable of defending himself against the things that he imagines are threatening him, such as bugs, rats, and snakes.

The room of such a patient should be lighted sufficiently so that shadows do not appear. Objects in the area should be well enough illuminated that they are not mistaken for other things. The patient's inner life is in a state of gross upheaval. He is frightened of his internal experiences and unable to trust his perceptions of the world surrounding him. It is comforting to the patient to find the external situation controlled by someone else in such a way that it is consistent and unwavering.

Occasionally, the adult patient becomes so extremely angry that he erupts combatively. This does not happen frequently, but when it does, it can usually be demonstrated that caregiving personnel did not pick up cues from the patient's verbal communication that he was annoyed or angry. These feelings were ignored or denied. Feelings that find no outlet are prone to grow, to become more inflammatory under pressure, and to explode. Though this kind of behavior is more often observed in children, it is well to remember that the hospitalized patient is encouraged to regress, to become more dependent and childlike. As he regresses psychologically, his physical responses can parallel this trend.

Mr. W., a 54-year-old German refugee, was admitted to the medical service with a diagnosis of osteogenic sarcoma. He was quite ill but had not been told his diagnosis or prognosis. Mr. W. had been interned in a concentration camp during the Second World War. The nurses observed that Mr. W. spoke adequate English but socialized little. His wife, who managed their small store during Mr. W.'s absence, spent much time at the bedside. The interviewer first became acquainted with Mr. W. when the staff nurses reported that he threw his water glass, full pitcher, tray, and full urinal into the hall at a passing nurse. When questioned, the floor nurses described this man as a person who became easily irritated. He was prone to frustration, communicated little, and was markedly uncooperative with the nurses. Only one male attendant was able to spend extended periods of time in the patient's room. Mr. W. seemed able to tolerate him.

Because of the nature of the nursing problem, a ward conference was held with the full staff present. From various descriptions of this patient's behavior, we decided that his combativeness was prompted by inordinate fear. We hypothesized that Mr. W.'s incarceration during the war had traumatized him so severely that his perception of the hospital and the people in it was grossly distorted. It seemed likely that Mr. W. perceived the nurses and doctors as sadistic, unreasonable authorities and that his enforced passive position made him feel unusually vulnerable to attack.

The nursing care plan centered on the key issue of Mr. W.'s overwhelming fears. The orderly was chosen to give Mr. W. most of his care in order that this patient could form one trusting relationship. The staff tried to communicate to him in every way possible that they were not cold, authoritative people but concerned, warm human beings. This was done by anticipating his needs, answering his light promptly, and sitting in the room whenever possible. Standing at the foot of the bed while conversing was discouraged, because this made the nurse appear taller—higher—than the patient. When the nurses were seated beside him, Mr. W. had the advantage of height.

Mr. W. responded favorably to these measures. Though he never became really talkative with the staff or verbalized his actual fears, the combative behavior ceased and the patient was discharged without further incidents.

Behavior that is unexpected or contrary to acceptable standards is frightening. The staff tends to withdraw from patients who frighten them. This is a poor situation. If some member of the staff can try to intervene by looking for *reasons* for the frightening behavior so that it may be understood, the behavior can be modified, and the staff can allay their anxieties before mutual withdrawal takes place.

BIBLIOGRAPHY

KRONER, K: *Dealing with the confused patient.* Nurs '79 9:71, 1979.
LETCHER, P, ET AL: *Reality orientation: A historical study of patient progress.* Hosp Community Psychiatry 25:801, 1974.

7

The Depressed Patient

Lisa Robinson, R.N., Ph.D., F.A.A.N., C.S.

The depressed patient can usually be diagnosed without difficulty. He is the individual who looks dejected and sad. He may cry often for no apparent reason. The depressed patient is quiet, perhaps even mute. Painful or distressing treatments provoke little reaction. The patient appears resigned to his fate. Often he does not eat. Sleeping patterns may also show disruption. The patient may be awake after two or three o'clock in the morning. The depressed patient who sleeps well all night sometimes experiences difficulty around the waking hour. This may be demonstrated by an inability to wake up and tend to the early morning washing before breakfast. Depression may be observed in the patient who cries upon awakening or in the patient who, upon arising, greets the unprepared nurse with numerous complaints about trivial issues. The basic problem is likely to be that the patient, already depressed and overwhelmed, awakens from sleep to find himself in the same dilemmas that he faced the previous day. Or, the depressed patient may sleep all day as a means of escaping depressing reality. Weight loss and constipation are additional indications of affective disorder.

More difficult to detect is depression in patients who mask their condition with somatic symptoms. These are the patients who develop headache or back pain or some other elusive complaint. The patient does not experience marked change in affect until the physical symptom, or depressive equivalent, is successfully treated, that is to say, until the physical symptom disappears. This type of patient is clinically depressed; however, the presence of the physical symptom staves off overt psychopathology.

The patient who becomes depressed while in the hospital is reacting to his situation in the same manner that he would no matter what the stress, be it illness, business failure, or misadventure. The individual responds to stimuli in a rather predictable manner. Past conflicts and solutions in the form of defenses provide the background for the patient's interpretation of his present experience and those factors that provide stress.

Patients who are candidates for mutilating surgery, such as radical cancer operations, are likely to experience depressive reactions postoperatively. They are faced not only with the preoperative anxiety that most surgical patients experience but also the overwhelming apprehension connected with the knowledge that they have carcinoma.[1,2] If a malignant neoplasm is not the reason for surgery, these patients must nonetheless face the fact that before they are anesthetized they are whole, but that some type of dismemberment will be performed on them before they are awakened. Postoperatively, these patients do tend to cope with the anxieties that arose before surgery and to come to terms with the images of their mutilated bodies. In the meantime, however, there may be some degree of transient depression.

The likelihood of such a response is influenced by the patient's preoperative personality and his anxiety. The prospect of surgery involves a real threat of danger. The threat lies, first, in the anesthesia and, second, in the actual operative procedure. The patient is forced to cope with the threat of extinction when he is put to sleep. Symbolically, being anesthetized is nonexistence, or death. Surgical intervention itself is perceived as a violation of body integrity and a violent attack.

Also a certain amount of suffering is realistically anticipated. Pain cannot be prepared for. The patient can only anticipate the physical sensation by recalling his responses to previous discomfort. Pain, as an event, is not recalled. It is the *feelings* about the event which remain vivid in memory. An example of this is the multipara who is anticipating delivery. She remembers previous labors and because of them does not look forward to the labor or delivery experience. However, her memories are actually of her fear and general inability to stem her discomfort; the sensation of pain itself is momentary.

The situation of the patient facing mutilating surgery is similar. He cannot prepare to cope with pain. He can only be aware of its eventuality and hope for support from internal strengths as well as medicinal intervention. Anxiety is engendered. Some patients will cope with it by becoming depressed.

Another unknown in the patient's ruminations is the chance for cure. It is well to sacrifice a part of one's body in order to preserve life, although this in itself is a most dire decision to make. However, to submit to mutilation in the *hope* of cure is even more traumatizing. The patient must face not only the loss of body integrity but the possibility of annihilation from the disease in spite of surgical intervention. All these factors in the patient's thinking influence the likelihood of postoperative depression.

The patient's attitude toward the affected organ is an important factor also. It is significant for its realistic and symbolic meaning. This is demonstrated repeatedly by patients who become depressed after minor gynecological procedures. The woman who is admitted for a dilatation and curettage may experience a reactive depression of the same magnitude as her roommate who has undergone a total abdominal hysterectomy. The reproductive organs are of great import to each individual, and their dysfunction and treatment engender anxiety. The genitals and breasts are important both symbolically and realistically to the woman. Her sexual identity revolves about these areas. Gynecological surgery carries its own special meaning, which influences depression.

The influence of the affected organ in depression is seen in the case of a 57-year-old man who had undergone an elective anal rectoplasty because of hemorrhoids. Postoperatively he would not feed himself, and his words were produced slowly and laboriously. After several days, the patient seemed less retarded. He reported to the nurses that he had felt infinitely sad and that he was apprehensive lest he never regain the ability to void normally or have a bowel movement. As these functions returned, the patient brightened considerably.

The patient undergoing mutilating surgery and the patient preparing for surgery on a highly significant organ come face to face with thoughts of pain, mutilation, and death. He must also confront the alteration of his body image. The laryngectomized patient awakens from surgery without a voice. He finds a hole in his neck with a piece of metal in it. He hears his breath whistling in and out of the aperture. He cannot produce sound. The patient recovering from a colon resection discovers his stool running out of a hole in his abdomen. All his childhood prohibitions are re-experienced. The sight and smell of feces make him feel dirty and ashamed. He wants desperately to control the stool but cannot. The patient with a radical mastectomy or limb amputation realizes the visible loss of a body part. The self-image is shattered. The person must become reacquainted with his own body whose very outline is changed. In each of these instances the patient must cope with extremely shocking reality factors postoperatively.

Chronic illnesses are sometimes accompanied by depression. Patients afflicted with such diseases as cancer, multiple sclerosis, poorly controlled diabetes, or tuberculosis may exist for an indeterminate length of time in a weakened and debilitated condition. Patients convalescing from myocardial infarctions or those who are cardiac invalids and are chronically ill also may become chronically depressed. Their illnesses mean, in many cases, the loss of gainful employment, the inability to guide a growing family, and the loss of identity as a strong, independent person. In addition, experiences that were once pleasurable may be impossible for the chronically ill patient.

In chronic illness, the patient realizes upon awakening each morning that the disease is unaltered. Perhaps a grave prognosis is threatening. The active, productive character who appeared in nighttime fantasy becomes the same sick, helpless, resigned person who awakens each day and discovers that wish-fulfilling dreams are fleeting. The long tedious hours of illness are constant.

The chronically ill patient who becomes depressed struggles with his inner world. He attempts to cope with frustration, helplessness, and hopelessness. He has been oppressed by loss of self-esteem and positive body image. He has been unable to control the invasion of his body by a disease process.

The following case demonstrates the problem of a depressed patient. Mrs. B., 36 years old and a mother and housewife, was admitted to the medical service for a fever of unknown origin. At the time, she reported feeling "too weak to pick up the coffee pot." She was hospitalized for diagnostic tests. After she had been in the hospital two weeks, none of the tests had revealed the cause of her elevated temperature.

The interviewer was asked to see this woman because of her numerous crying spells and general depression. She was in bed eating breakfast when the interviewer met her. The patient began to cry immediately, saying that she was so unhappy, she had been hospitalized for two weeks and wanted to go home. She complained that numerous blood samples had been drawn and that blood had been left on her sheets and that she was afraid. She continued saying that she was to have a blood transfusion and was terribly afraid of that too. When asked if she had ever had one before, she said that many years before, when she had had subacute bacterial endocarditis, she had been transfused. She related also that when she had had her baby, she had been given sodium Pentothal, which, though her doctor did not know it, she was allergic to, and that she had become quite ill. Without transition, she continued that she was afraid, she hated to see sick people in the hospital, and she thought that she would never get well. If only she could go home she would surely recover. Mrs. B. then launched into a discussion of her children and how much she wanted to see them. She knew she could get permission for the younger child to come into the hospital, but she did not want to do this because it would mean that she was not going to go home and become well again.

From the material presented, the interviewer saw Mrs. B. as an overconcerned, worrying patient. She sounded anxious and phobic about medical procedures. Her behavior indicated some depressive feelings. With this type of patient, each potentially threatening situation might be linked with an increased variety of old anxieties stemming mainly from childhood. The patient's main problems often stem from a learned behavioral response that results in a feeling of helplessness. In earlier years, the ego was too weak to tolerate the onslaught of anxiety and in response to such stress, the individual learned to feel and to be helpless. In adulthood, although other behavioral responses to stress are available, the individual unconsciously selects the anxiety → helplessness → depression triad. From this ego state, current imagined dangers are almost always far more threatening than reality.

Mrs. B. responded well to a nursing care plan that included giving her the feeling of being protected by a strong, knowledgeable, helpful person. The facts concerning her illness were discussed in simple, appropriate, and comprehensible form as she initiated conversation about them. The rationale of her treatment and of the expected cure was explained. Vague and frightening formulations were avoided. Superfluous information was not divulged, since Mrs. B. could not readily assimilate it. When possible, Mrs. B. was placed in situations that she could control. In other words, she was helped to feel less like a helpless child.

Mrs. S. was an apprehensive patient who had been admitted for an axillary node biopsy. Several x-ray studies were done. One series required that the patient fast prior to the test. The nurses explained to Mrs. S. the reason that her meal trays were being withheld. The patient said nothing; however, upon her return from Radiology, she went to the telephone booth and called her husband. The nurses heard Mrs. S. commanding him to come get her immediately. She told Mr. S. that she was being starved. The husband apparently placated her. Her behavior, however, made the nurses feel anxious.

I met Mrs. S. the next day. The patient seemed in good control and we chatted briefly. I told Mrs. S. I would see her the following Monday.

After the weekend, I went to the unit and discovered that Mrs. S. had undergone a radical mastectomy over the weekend. (The tests had indicated a need for immediate surgical intervention.) Mrs. S. was propped up in bed, she was receiving intravenous fluids, and looked quite ill.

I approached Mr. S., saying, "What a surprise. So much has happened to you since my last visit."

"Yes," answered the patient, smiling unconvincingly, "my husband hurt his leg Saturday." (This was true.) We spoke briefly, and I promised to return the following day. Mrs. S. was seen for five days consecutively. She continued to remain in bed, cried each day, and

moved about only after much encouragement. During this peri
Mrs. S. wore no cosmetics and her personal hygiene was poor.

In conference with the staff nurses, we decided that Mrs. S. was depressed. She had, of course, very reality-based reasons for her depression. The staff reviewed Mrs. S.'s hospital course. She had been extremely anxious prior to surgery. This was demonstrated substantially by her inability to comprehend the nurse's explanation of the x-ray studies. The surgical procedure had been done rather suddenly. It was hypothesized that Mrs. S., already incapacitated by anxiety, was unable to marshall her defenses in order to buffer her ego against further stress related to the surgery. In her remarks about her husband's injury on the Monday following her operation, she demonstrated the use of denial in an effort to adjust to the severe trauma she had experienced. This denial was unproductive, however, because it did not help her to get the active support she was in need of.

The nursing care plan that was devised allowed this patient much time and opportunity to discuss her surgery and to explore with the nurse its actual meaning and consequences. The plan permitted Mrs. S. to exist temporarily in a highly structured environment. Eating, bathing, ambulating, and even applying makeup were made into a schedule. Along with consistent encouragement to handle these activities herself, Mrs. S. was given a great deal of attention. She was praised for her appearance, her discrimination in selecting clothes to wear, her cooperation, and so on. The nurses communicated their hearty approval of this patient as a woman.

By the sixth postoperative day, Mrs. S. was up and about without encouragement. She was taking full responsibility for her personal hygiene, including her normal attention to cosmetics. She had been able to discuss her operation in realistic terms.

In summary, when dealing with the chronically ill patient or the postoperative patient who is depressed, the nurse needs to realize that there is intrapsychic meaning in the patient's situation. In the case of the chronically ill patient, it is well to consider the meaning and impact of the disease. Though often he is not aware of it, the symbolic meaning influences his thoughts and behavior. The careful listener can learn about her patient's unconscious thoughts by being

ice of conversational topics, descriptive words, and
rsing care. To share these observations with the pa-
ssary; indeed, it is contraindicated in the majority of
nursing care can be planned in such a way as to
...e patient to come to terms with his feelings.

The nurse who is permissive and nonjudgmental gives her patient
the opportunity to discuss his thoughts and feelings. His seemingly
irrational anger and hostile fantasies can be expressed without fear of
retaliation. The smoldering resentment that the patient may feel toward a "sadistic" surgeon or "brutal" nurses can be verbalized
openly, so that anxiety need not later be the cause of a reactive depression.

The perceptive nurse can manage her patient's needs therapeutically if she can find ways to allow him choices in his daily living. If
hopefulness and means of self-fulfillment can be maintained in the
patient, his life can have meaning and purpose. Maneuvers such as
allowing him to choose his own menus, plan his own time for morning care, or decide when to get out of his room for a trip to the solarium are means of providing the patient with some control of his own
affairs.

The nurse caring for a patient who is a potential candidate for depression must exercise her ingenuity. She needs to be aware that
there are underlying feelings such as anger, guilt, or anxiety. These
emotions are part of the patient's personality. Though the basic problems of the depressed patient will probably not come to light during
the hospitalization, the nurses can assist him by modifying his environment and making personnel available for communication. It is not
useful to the patient for the nurse to ignore the depression or attempt
to modify it by enticement or admonishment. Sitting with the patient,
saying little or nothing, and maintaining a matter-of-fact or neutral
attitude are helpful. This permits the patient to talk if he wishes, to
complain if he so desires, or to respond in whatever manner is indicated by his intrapsychic processes rather than by the dictates of a
social situation.

REFERENCES

1. BRESSLER, B, COHEN, S, AND MAGNUSSEN, F: *The problem of phantom breast and phantom pain.* J Nerv Ment Dis 123:181, 1956.
2. BARD, M AND SUTHERLAND, A: *Psychological impact of cancer and its treatment. Adaptation to radical mastectomy.* Cancer 8:656, 1955.

BIBLIOGRAPHY

DEUTSCH, H: *Some psychoanalytic observations in surgery.* Psychosom Med 4:105, 1942.

GRINKER, R, ET AL: *The Phenomena of Depression.* Harper & Row, New York, 1961.

HACKETT, TP AND WEISMAN, A: *Psychiatric management of operative syndromes.* Psychosom Med 22:267, 1960.

KNOWLES, R: *Handling depression by identifying anger.* Am J Nurs 968, 1981.

_____: *Handling depression through activity.* Am J Nurs 81:1187, 1981.

_____: *Handling depression through positive reinforcement.* 81:1353, 1981.

LINDEMANN, E: *Observations on psychiatric sequelae to surgical operations in women.* Am J Psychiatry 98:132, 1941.

RUBIN, R: *Body image and self esteem.* Nurs Outlook 16:20, 1968.

UJHELY, G: *Grief and depression: Implications for prevention and therapeutic nursing care.* Nurs Forum 5:23, 1966.

8

The Demanding Patient

Lisa Robinson, R.N., Ph.D., F.A.A.N., C.S.

As has been previously discussed, nurses are motivated to enter their profession by various reasons. It is characteristic of people who decide to become nurses that they recognize and tolerate well the dependency needs of others. It can be observed that people who become nurses enjoy meeting these needs. They receive some gratification from nurturing those who require it.

Nurses see themselves as caregiving people. Others tend to identify nurses in a similar manner. It is an expectation of patients that the nurse will take care of them, that is, recognize their needs, gratify them, and thereby make them feel better. This expectation is also held by the nurse herself.

At times, the nurse's initial endeavors do not meet the patient's needs. The patient continues to feel physically uncomfortable or anxious or both. If the nurse is well motivated, she will make further efforts to intervene therapeutically. In most cases, if the nurse persists, she eventually makes her patient more comfortable.

Occasionally, the nurse does not discover a satisfactory solution for herself and the patient. The patient, who initiated the process by indicating a need for something, becomes frustrated. He may withdraw from the situation as a way of avoiding further conflict. He may react with anger or become more persistent in his demands upon the nurse, propelling himself into further conflict. The situation is rather analogous to that of two bulls who lock horns in combat. Neither participant in the battle can step back far enough to gain momentum

arge. So it is for the nurse and her patient. The nurse
to satisfy the demand. As her attempts to satisfy the
peatedly, she tends to become frustrated or angry or
... because of her heightened feelings, she becomes less organized, and thus, tends to be less effective in identifying and solving
the problem. Because of this, the nurse becomes repetitive, giving the
same type of response over and over again.

The patient becomes increasingly perturbed if his need is not ful-
filled. His emotional response is exaggerated. The nurse reacts to him
and his feelings. Anxiety is produced from the impasse (conflict). This
is the usual background situation when a patient is labeled demanding. The nurse has not met the patient's need. The patient's expectation of her as a nurturing person has not proven correct. The nurse's
expectation of the patient has, likewise, proven wrong—the patient
has not received the nurse's ministrations passively and with grateful
demeanor. In this situation, the roles have conflicted.

The solution to the problem lies in careful analysis of it. The basic
question to be answered is "What does the patient *really* want?" If the
nurse has responded to the patient's overt request and the patient
continues to call upon her, then it may be assumed that the patient
needs something that has not been stated. It is then incumbent on the
nurse to attempt to identify the latent components of the patient's
demands.

To be effective, the nurse must be relatively free of anxiety so that
she can explore the situation. That is to say, the nurse must be sufficiently free of potentially disorganizing feelings to be able to channel
her resources into this constructive pursuit.

The ability to control her own anxiety will permit the nurse to scrutinize her reaction to the patient. She can focus on her own feelings
when the patient does not respond appropriately or as anticipated.
This may involve becoming aware of her irritation or anger at the
demanding patient. She must be sufficiently aware of her own feelings to separate her subjective evaluation of the patient (which may
be colored by frustration, annoyance, or anger) from how the patient
actually presents himself.

Having identified her own feelings about the patient, the nurse can
formulate her profile of him and his problem more objectively. If she
is particularly attuned to her own feelings, she can use herself as a

sort of barometer. She can take a reading on the emotional climate she finds herself in with her patient. That is to say, if the nurse is working with a patient who seems too sweet and patronizing, and there is something that cannot quite be identified, the nurse might find herself reacting with inexplicable annoyance or, more forcefully, with anger. This provides a clue to the nurse. What is it in her relationship with this patient that is stimulating her to be angry? The nurse can then go back and scrutinize the patient more closely. Perhaps the patient is rather hostile and is hiding his feelings behind a facade of sweetness. Perhaps the patient is really quite angry and trying to cope with these feelings.

At times, female patients feel competitive with their nurses. This type of situation arises in cases where a female patient is basically unsure of herself as a feminine person and needs again and again to gain masculine approval. The doctor takes on a role of a potentially approving male as well as the healing person. He is also, within the hospital environment, comparable to the father. The nurses are perceived (unconsciously) as mother figures or sibling rivals. The patient, then, is attempting to gain the approval of the doctor. The nurses who work closely with the doctor are seen by the patient as rivals for his attention and are treated with some hostility by the patient.

This is a potentially explosive situation. The patient, in an attempt to establish a closer relationship with the doctor, may set up a triangle and make the nurses the scapegoats. Another possible triangle involves the nurses scapegoating the patient and drawing closer to the doctor. Still a third possibility is for the doctor to initiate the scapegoating. In any of these cases, everyone involved is penalized. The situation must be explored through objective data so that the patient's needs can be identified. It is equally important that the doctor's and nurses' needs for recognition and esteem be gratified through appropriate channels.

This kind of situation is rarely experienced at a conscious level by either the patient or the nurse. It can be picked up by the astute nurse who correctly identifies her own feelings toward the patient and works back to the sources of these feelings.

The patient who makes numerous requests of the nurse when he could conceivably be helping himself, or the patient who makes numerous requests of the nurse who has attempted unsuccessfully to respond to his requests, is usually labeled demanding. His demand-ingness is an attempt to make himself feel better. To understand what is making this patient feel uncomfortable, one needs to scrutinize the results of his behavior. The demanding patient receives attention. The attention he gets from nurses, relatives, and friends means security to him. It is not far afield to assume that the demanding patient, that is, the patient whose verbalized needs have been met but who persists in making demands upon the nurse, is actually trying to gain *security*.

The next step in analyzing the problem is to look at the possible reasons for the patient's particular need for security at this time. Per-haps the patient is afraid, and the repeated appearances of a nurse are reassuring. Perhaps he is very lonely but thinks it ridiculous to di-vulge these thoughts. Such a theory may merit consideration if the nurse recalls with honesty how many patients have called her into their rooms in a given week and requested her to keep them company because they were lonely. Perhaps the patient equates attention with approval.

A 67-year-old woman, hospitalized for gastrointestinal bleeding, was a constant source of irritation to the nurses. She required expert nursing care because she was quite ill. Her bowels were loose and often bloody. She could not control these massive evacuations and soiled the bed often. The nurses cleaned and changed her whenever necessary. Despite these attentions, the patient was constantly whin-ing and making demands on the staff. She clung to them when they were near her bed and tried to ingratiate herself with them.

As I listened to this patient's monologue, I noted that the woman talked about her soiling repetitively, saying many times that she could not control it. These comments were interwoven with physical com-plaints and bids for further attention. I pointed out that the nurses knew that the patient could not control her soiling and that they truly wanted to be helpful. I reassured the patient that the nurses would not leave her in a dirty bed and added that these loose bowel move-ments must be terribly difficult to contend with, and that the nurses knew what a struggle it was for the patient and were sympathetic. These comments were echoed by the nurses who cared for her.

The patient's behavior did not change radically, but there was less comment about her diarrhea and her efforts to be ingratiating were not as noticeable. As with all extremely demanding patients, it was necessary to try to understand the real nature of the requests made. This woman was quite ill. Many of her demands were indisputably legitimate. An equal number were seemingly pointless and very annoying to the nurses—her clinging to them physically, her fawning comments, and her excessive requests of the nurses when they were in her room.

It seemed that this patient wanted to keep the staff with her constantly. She literally held them; she made comments designed to flatter and keep the nurses' attention. She contrived all kinds of tasks that would keep personnel around her.

Why did she want or need the nurses around her constantly? Was she frightened, lonely, in pain? Possibly all three assumptions were correct; however, the patient herself gave clues to the meaning of her behavior. She kept reiterating in her conversations that she could not control her stool. She seemed, in effect, to be trying to justify her predicament to those caring for her. It was as if she felt their disapproval. My comments were in response to these declamations.

The nurses denied disapproval of their patient's incontinence or thoughts of punitive actions toward her. Subsequently, the patient did not focus on this area, so it can be assumed that this was a reasonable interpretation of the problem. Her response gave further credence to the assumption that the patient found herself repugnant in the throes of her illness and projected these attitudes onto those caring for her. Of course, it should be kept in mind that the nurses *had* been annoyed at the patient's general behavior. This lady may well have sensed their irritation and attributed it to her loss of control of her bowels. No matter how the problem arose or in what order its elements were solved, the patient did respond to the appropriate type of attention. Her anxiety was alleviated when the nurses communicated their approval of the patient and their awareness that she could not control her soiling of the bed.

Generally speaking, the demanding patient is a person who is lonely, frightened, or anxious. Sometimes the demanding patient holds himself in very low esteem. He often assumes that others regard him similarly. The demanding patient's multitudinous requests for water, bedpan, straightened draw sheet, and other minutiae can be bids for attention that are equivalent to bids for security and reassurance. When the nurse gives the appropriate type of attention, she is communicating the idea that even though the individual (patient) may not be acceptable to himself (may have a poor self-image), he can still receive attention (approval, recognition) from the nurses.

The validity of the nurse's interpretation of the problem can be judged by the patient's behavior. If it is altered, then something has happened between the patient and the nurse. It is likely that the nurse has given the patient sufficient support to feel less threatened.

This kind of nursing intervention is most effectively done in many short visits, rather than one long encounter. The nurse meets the patient's need for support by coming in the room and seating herself comfortably for at least five or ten minutes. She is more effective if she can convey to the patient that she truly wishes to spend the time in this manner and that she is not rushing to get away. If the nurse tells her patient as she leaves the room when she plans to return, and if the nurse keeps her word, the patient is likely to be less active in the use of the bell cord.

Mrs. Y., a 62-year-old widow, came to the hospital because she had pneumonia. As soon as she was admitted, Mrs. Y. made her presence known to all. Her complaints were loud and numerous. After several days of verbal abuse, the staff nurses requested consultation.

They reported that if Mrs. Y. was not given complete morning care first thing in the morning she complained vigorously. If her roommate was visited by a nurse, Mrs. Y. wondered verbally and with indignation why she was not accorded the same treatment. She refused her food, saying it was vile. Her opinion of the nursing care was given freely. She found it abominable.

When I first saw Mrs. Y., I found her curled up in her disheveled bed. I drew the curtains around the unit, asking if I might visit with Mrs. Y. After a brief introduction, I sat back and let Mrs. Y. enumerate the many indignities she had suffered. The patient said the nursing care was terrible. She would have done better staying at home. She had lost her husband one year before this hospitalization and now lived with her daughter, who cared for her "much better than these nurses." This statement was repeated several times. In an angry tirade, this little elderly lady said that she could not afford to contribute $5000 to the hospital, but that she still ought to have some care. At one point Mrs. Y. said, "I am not scum. I should not be treated this way." She cried bitterly. I remained with Mrs. Y. for quite a while and when I left, promised to return the next morning.

In a ward conference, the staff nurses all described similar experiences with Mrs. Y. One nurse recalled that Mrs. Y.'s roommate could always predict how bad the day would be for Mrs. Y. by how she awoke in the morning. It was theorized that Mrs. Y. was severely regressed, depressed, and in need of special care. One of the particularly pertinent clues to Mrs. Y.'s feelings was the way she presented herself on arising in the morning. As has been described, patients who are depressed often find the morning hours especially horrendous. Mrs. Y.'s comments led the staff to believe that she viewed herself as a worthless individual who was helpless. She saw the situation as one in which her fate was in the hands of nurses who did not care about her. It seemed to her that her only salvation lay in the hands of various important people in her life who she assumed "would not tolerate this situation if they knew about it." She never indicated any confidence in her own ability to alter her situation.

The nurses decided to visit Mrs. Y. first thing each morning after the change-of-shift conference. One of them would wake her up with a cup of hot coffee and sit with her while she drank it. If time was available, she would be given her bath. If not, Mrs. Y.'s care would be deferred until after breakfast. The key issue was sitting with Mrs. Y. and explaining the situation to her. Later each morning she would be wheeled to the solarium and given the newspaper. Several visits would be made to her room during the day for conversations of five or ten minutes' duration. At least once an hour, a nurse would check with the patient to see if anything was desired.

The patient did nicely on this regimen. Her complaints decreased in number and loudness. She became so attached to one of the nurses that she insisted on the nurse's accepting the gift of a box of powder. The nurse, wisely, did not refuse. Though this was ignoring a specific hospital policy, the nurse realized that Mrs. Y. felt important and autonomous in extending this token of her appreciation and that its refusal would have hurt the patient deeply.

The following case illustrates the technique of behavior modification. Additionally, many theories were offered concerning the patient's behavior, upon which a nursing care plan was structured.

Though the constructs were never validated, the outcome of the work was good.

A request for consultation was received from the surgical service concerning a 28-year-old divorced barmaid who had been on the ward for one month prior to the consultation. She had been admitted for an ischiorectal abscess. The history showed that she had ulcerative colitis and was on a maintenance dose of steroids. There had been periodic flare-ups of her disease in the past five years. Also it was noted that the patient had an "alcohol problem."

The request for consultation was made because the patient was so demanding. Soon after her admission, her abscess had been drained in the operating room under general anesthesia. The area was packed and the patient returned to the floor. Immediately she began to cause a severe commotion on the ward. She whined and cried constantly and told the nurses that she could not get out of bed because her knees were too weak and her pain too great. Indeed the patient's physical condition was not good. She remained febrile and was nauseated much of the time. For some time she was fed intravenously and for a portion of that period she received hyperalimentation.

When the consultant saw T.W. there was a definite disparity between the perceptions of staff and those of the consultant concerning the patient's level of behavior. Staff characterized her as extremely infantile, whining and moaning continuously, claiming that she could not move because of her intense pain. They said she began to cry as soon as someone entered her room, and this behavior was driving staff away from her.

When the consultant entered T.W.'s room, the patient was lying on her side talking to a man who stood by the bedside. Another man was in her adjoining bathroom. The door to this room was ajar, affording a glimpse of the man shaving. When the consultant entered and introduced herself, T.W. offered the information that the man beside her was her former husband and the man in the bathroom was one of her boyfriends. T.W. spoke in a soft, well modulated voice. She gave no evidence of the histrionics described by staff.

The consultant addressed all three in the room, saying that she was there to help T.W. plan for her care. She said the nurses were concerned that T.W. was not out of bed often enough for her wound to heal satisfactorily and they wondered if T.W. could help schedule a plan that would be both comfortable and useful. The patient listened attentively but said nothing. The consultant, having stated her business, said she would return later when T.W. did not have company. The consultant reported to the staff how surprised she felt at the maturity of T.W.'s behavior in the company of her ex-husband and boyfriend. Because of this potential, the consultant decided with the staff to try to provide incentives for this level of behavior rather than the infantile behavior that was seen in the absence of her male company.

It was observed by staff that T.W. often cried for her mother. At the same time, the patient reported that she and her mother did not get along well and that, actually, she was quite *afraid* of her. It was conjectured that since T.W. and her mother seemed to have a rather disturbed relationship, perhaps the patient transferred much of her feelings for her mother to the nurses who were also giving her mothering care, and that perhaps her behavior represented her ambivalence toward her mother. Staff felt that her continuous crying and calling them was designed to bring them to her (at the conscious level), while her obnoxious behavior acted to drive them away (unconsciously). Because of her completely different behavior with men, as observed by the consultant, it was felt that there was some evidence that T.W. found it easier to relate to the opposite sex.

Based on this theory, it was decided to rotate staff caring for T.W. so that no one had to deal too long with negative feelings in response to the patient's provocative behavior. In addition, the plan allowed T.W. sufficient distance from individual nurses so that the troublesome mother-child type of relationship did not develop. If the theory about her behavior was valid, T.W.'s stress would be lessened.

One of the staff was to see her at least once every half hour. Directions were to be given matter-of-factly and negative behavior was not to be accepted. Thus, if the patient was asked to get out of bed, the nurse was not to accept a no answer. The patient would either get up unassisted, or she would be gotten out of bed. When she did well, T.W. was to be praised.

The consultant went back to the patient. She explained to T.W. that in order for her wound to heal the patient needed to get out of bed to increase the blood circulation to the wound in order to bring to the tissue those elements needed for healing. T.W. was gotten up by the consultant and then shown how to feel her own pulse in order to know the effect of activity on her heart beat, that is, on her circulation. T.W. told the consultant that she longed to talk to her mother. She described at length positive feelings for this woman. Because of the report, the consultant decided to use the mother-child relationship as incentive for the patient to follow the treatment regimen. She told T.W. that when she could tolerate sitting up in a chair long enough, she could be wheeled to the phone to call her mother. That was the first goal. Second, the consultant pointed out that the daily calls to her mother via the wheelchair might then be replaced by walks to the phone and soon after that, the patient would be well enough to walk out of the hospital. The patient seemed enthusiastic. Consultant and patient made a chart upon which the patient was to write for each session out of bed the number of minutes she was able to tolerate being up. The patient was instructed that the staff would not insist on a particular time but that they would assist T.W. to get up twice a day, and it was her responsibility to lengthen the time as she felt able.

Initially, the consultant worked with T.W. getting her out of bed. The patient whined and complained that her legs would not hold her up. She said she could not feel her legs under her and that she was scared. (Staff had described this type of behavior and said the patient would slump to the floor and refuse to get up, saying she was unable.) The consultant worked by placing her hands on the patient's knees and instructing her to lock them under the hands of the nurse. The patient complied and was turned around so that she could swing from the bed immediately into the chair behind her. She was given the consultant's watch and told that perhaps 10 to 15 minutes would be a good starting interval for the patient's self-directed therapy. Conversation was made, focusing on the patient's courage while attempting a painful but necessary treatment. When the patient noted that five minutes had passed and she could not tolerate more, T.W. was immediately helped back to bed.

The consultant was concerned with the patient's description of her lack of feeling in her legs and looked through the chart for any evidence to suggest a neurological deficit. The notes described an incidence of "shock" as the result of allergic response to the hyperalimentation; however, a neurological examination had been done and the conclusion was that there was no demonstrable evidence of lesion.

The daily work with T.W. continued. She did not like getting up but did so when she was told matter-of-factly that it was necessary. When she threatened to fall to the floor, it was pointed out that the floor was dirty and her incision might become infected if she did this. T.W. was praised for her efforts in getting into the chair. Although staff did try to prolong her out-of-bed intervals, they abided by her wishes when she said she could not stand being up any longer.

T.W. extended her time out of bed very slowly. Though her physical condition improved, the patient's mental set seemed to reflect her ambivalence about getting well and leaving the hospital. It was obvious to the staff that she was not in any hurry to go. Finally, however, T.W. could not deny that her wound was healed, she could ambulate comfortably, and no matter what her social and familial problems were, she had to leave the hospital and face them.

BIBLIOGRAPHY

BRACELAND, F: *Loneliness—Man's universal plaint*. In SIPE, AWR (ED): *Hope*. Brunner/Mazel, New York, 1970.

FROMM-REICHMANN, F: *On loneliness*. In BULLARD, D (ED): *Psychoanalysis and Psychotherapy*. University of Chicago Press, Chicago, 1959.

KING, J: *A therapeutic approach to acting out and its ramifications*. In DUFFEY, M, ET AL (EDS): *Current Concepts in Clinical Nursing, Vol III*. CV Mosby, St. Louis, 1971.

PREDDY, E: *Mutual hostility—That was the risk with Mark*. Nurs '75 1:13, 1975.

9
The Chronically Ill Patient

Lisa Robinson, R.N., Ph.D., F.A.A.N., C.S.

The age of technology has brought many valuable innovations and discoveries to the world. Improved contraception, trips to outer space, and new forms of energy are all by-products of 20th century science; increased life span is yet another. The last presents both advantages and liabilities. With increased longevity goes a higher incidence of chronic diseases. These include heart conditions, arthritis and rheumatism, impairments of lower extremities and hips, visual impairments, and hypertension without heart involvement. Also, because of medical advances, diseases that were once acute and quickly terminal can now be altered to a chronic status. Among these are such problems as renal failure, some of the leukemias and other blood dyscrasias, collagen diseases, and diabetes.

The Commission on Chronic Illness (1956) defined chronic illness as:

> All impairments or deviations from normal which have one or many of the following characteristics: are permanent, leave residual disability, are caused by non-reversible pathological alteration, require special training of the patient for rehabilitation, may be expected to require a long period of supervision, observation, or care.[1]

The advantages of longer life are easily recognized by all those who enjoy it; the liabilities are often not as obvious to those who do not suffer from chronic diseases. Basically, it is the *quality* of life that may be severely impaired. To persons who are restricted to a bed or whose lives depend on the running of a machine with intercurrent periods of intense pain, anxiety, and physiological complications, and to those who struggle for each lungful of air, the liabilities of longevity are known.

Persons who suffer from chronic diseases must live differently from the way they lived prior to their symptoms. Movement may present insurmountable problems. The need for a wheelchair may mean no trips to the movies or theater or even no shopping. Dressing and undressing when desired may be a luxury that is not affordable, because arthritic fingers cannot grasp buttons or zippers. Trips outside of the home may have to be carefully planned, based on the ability of the chronically ill person to rest and renew his oxygen supply. Holding a job and joining friends for social occasions may be precluded by either the person's impairment or the unpredictable return of symptoms.

The chronically ill are known to health care providers because of their need for maintenance of prescribed treatment, prevention or management of medical crises, control of symptoms, and adjustment to changes in the course of the disease through exacerbations and remissions.[2]

The chronically ill person is a patient very different from the acutely ill individual. The latter is typically naive about his condition and its treatment. Entry into the health care system is frightening, because the acutely ill patient does not know what to expect. This patient is socialized into the role of patient. Other patients and staff quickly communicate the health care system's expectations of the patient role and the acutely ill person conforms. He becomes passive, sometimes regresses to earlier coping behaviors, depends heavily on physician, nurses, and family for need fulfillment, and does whatever is asked in the way of cooperation with health care providers. Typically, this patient has faith in his doctor and thinks that the illness will be successfully treated and the prior health status will be regained.

For the chronically ill patient, few of these statements pertain. The person with a long-term illness usually knows the health care system intimately. He is also known by that system. Patients and staff have rigid expectations of each other's behavior. The patient may know that his clinic doctor will tell him how irresponsible he is as soon as the patient's weight is read from the chart. The female patient may know that the nurse who greets her in the OB clinic will say, "Why Rita Booth, I thought we told you not to get pregnant again. Don't you understand how your heart has to overwork?" A patient may also know that a clinic appointment for 9 A.M. means three buses and a wait of at least three hours before she sees the doctor. The patient may elect to leave the clinic before being seen, if the baby sitter cannot stay more than two and a half hours. Or if there is no baby sitter, the patient may leave without being seen because she is too worried about her toddlers to wait the requisite time.

The chronically ill patient has other knowledge also. He knows how it is to be sick all the time, how it is to be socially isolated because erstwhile friends don't want to take the time to come over because they are embarrassed about not knowing what to say, or because as their lives have unfolded they have moved on and no longer have things in common with the patient who has not enjoyed these progressions.

The patient knows how it is to be always waiting for the disease's next exacerbation, wondering what has caused it, and how it might have been prevented. The patient knows the trials and tribulations of looking for money to pay doctor bills, clinic bills, hospital bills, drug bills, and an endless stream of other bills. The patient knows a routine for maintaining his physiological stability. For example, the ostomy is irrigated at a certain time to prevent embarrassing accidents. Certain foods are avoided because they cause diarrhea or telltale gas.

There is also a routine for managing psychological stability. Implications of new symptoms may be denied. Anger at doctors and nurses is isolated from offensive events. Frustration with family is suppressed. Routines are rigidly adhered to. Many of these coping behaviors and defenses are violated by health care providers, because they do not understand their patients well enough to recognize the significance of observed behaviors. Because staff do not understand the ritual involved in a patient's dressing change, the former may deny the patient's security operation or they may discount his need for it. Staff may judge the patient incompetent, when actually he has done remarkably well by developing the stabilizing routine. While hospitalized, the patient may be infantilized, because he is denied the opportunity to do things that he is fully capable of doing for himself at home. On the other hand, staff may push a patient toward premature independence, not realizing that he is exhausted and needs to regress and to be temporarily granted dependent status. Because staff and patient may not take the time for meaningful dialogue, all parties may have different notions of the chronically ill patient's needs.

Ms. A. is a 28-year-old single woman who has moderately severe cerebral palsy. She has had multiple hospitalizations for correction of various problems. She is wheelchair bound and very demanding. Her urologist has brought her into the hospital for evaluation of complaints related to her ileostomy. The physician is unable to discover the cause of her complaints. The nurses want Ms. A. discharged, because she is not receiving treatment but is extremely demanding and requires extensive nursing assistance with activities of daily living. The patient believes that she has received nothing helpful from the hospitalization. She has tried repeatedly to get relief but no one seems to understand her. She complains to a sibling that life is not worth living, and she says that she is contemplating suicide.

The acutely ill patient is impaired for a short and predictable interval. Medical and nursing intervention typically addresses alteration of the disease process. Occasionally, psychological and social facets of the patient's existence are also examined. In the case of the chronically ill person it is imperative that the total patient be addressed, because the disease process affects all aspects of the patient's life and, like the disease, its effects are long-lived. Some of the crucial issues that are dealt with involve roles; passivity and activity are highly influenced by the disease process, the patient's strivings, and the expectations of significant others. Self-concept and self-esteem are altered by chronic illness. Social interaction is altered; some chronically ill patients must struggle to find a balance between total involvement with self and concern for others. Patients must often depend on family, significant others, or health care providers to meet their needs. Because of this necessary dependence, they are in conflict about expression of provocative feelings or thoughts. Daily irritations and frustrations may accumulate because they are not shared.

Mr. L., a fifty-year-old married man with four grown children, lives with his wife and one adult daughter. He was diagnosed with lymphoma 11 years ago. This patient has had several recent hospital admissions because his disease has progressed. (He now has nodes in his neck, and his right leg is painful.) The patient has had several rounds of chemotherapy. The most recent was one week ago. The patient has been seeking the attention of many of the ward staff and physicians making rounds. He appears anxious and tremulous. When one enterprising medical student finally takes the time to sit down and talk with this patient, he finds out that the patient over-heard the resident and attending physician say that Mr. L.'s chemo-therapy was "20 percent effective." No one has explained whether that means that he has 20 percent of the tumor left or whether that means that 20 percent has gone away. Mr. L. has been consumed with worry but unable to bring himself to seek clarification from his attending physician.

Some patients feel an intense desire to be cared for, but they know that others will not comply. They respond with feelings of intense anger.

Mr. B. is a 33-year-old black carpenter. He has chronic renal failure, cirrhosis of the liver, and hypertension. Mr. B. was promised during his admission that he would be dialyzed the next day and then he would be discharged and referred elsewhere for outpatient dialysis. The promised treatment did not materialize because of lack of coordi-nation with the department of urology. The patient has been incarcer-ated on many occasions, and he sees hospitalization as jail—a place where someone else has control and power over him. Mr. B. is very angry with his physicians whom he blames for not delivering what they promised. He does not accept bureaucratic obstructions as rea-sonable excuses for denial of his treatment and discharge.

Some patients allow themselves the luxury of expressing hostile feeling. They think, with some justification, that needed alliances with others will be destroyed by their apparent lack of gratitude. They become bitter and skeptical. They are often shunned by others.

The unit nurses have sought consultation with the psychiatric liai-son nurse. Their problem patient is Ms. V. who is hospitalized be-cause of sickle cell crisis. The patient, a 21-year-old black woman, has had the disease since age eight or nine. She has had three to four crises per year. According to the nurses, Ms. V. does not comply with her prescribed regimen. Currently the patient is separated from her husband. Their only child died in infancy from sickle cell disease. The nurses find it difficult to take care of this patient, because she "doesn't care enough to take care of herself."

On interview, the nurse hears that Ms. V. dreads coming back into the hospital. She knows that the staff do not like her. She cannot control her symptoms, and she knows that they cannot either. Ms. V. wonders why the staff expects her to be able to keep herself well, when they cannot make her well.

Another problem of the chronically ill is the stigma under which they live. Nurses and doctors and lay persons tend to prefer interacting with patients who are going to recover. It is depressing to be with someone who always has to struggle to live or with the patient whose downhill course is inexorable. So these patients become accustomed to being the last ones cared for. They are the patients who answer the visiting nurse's ring at 4:30 P.M. They are the patients who are set up for their baths by the aide and are told that she will be back sometime later in the morning after trays are collected. These patients grow accustomed to the meaningless "Hi, how are you?" from staff who wave from the doorway but never come in. They are used to meaningless chit-chat, because care providers do not know what to say. The chronically ill tend to be lonely, because they have become disenfranchised.

What can health care providers do to enrich the lives of their chronically ill patients? Obviously, their physical condition must be monitored and kept as close to normal as possible. The same might be said of their psychosocial conditions. These patients tend to have numerous problems in the psychosocial sphere that need attention. They need either jobs or tasks to use their skills. They need attention from other people who are not concerned primarily with their health. They need funds to pay for their material goods. They need a chance to get out of their rooms, to go to the movies, to attend an end-of-the-month sale. They need confidantes with whom to share. They need people to love. Nursing personnel are not always the most appropriate resources for meeting the chronically ill patient's needs, but they might be the only people who are around the patient enough to know what the patient needs. The best way to assess the patient's needs is to

listen to the patient and his family. They wil[...]
opportunity. Strauss and Glaser write:

> . . . the chronically ill (and their families) usua[...]
> to give those data. Many sick persons, as we h[...]
> able to tell other people about their difficulties[...]
> for a variety of reasons, and some suffer from[...]
> (The researchers) . . . discovered how eager [...]
> about themselves and their disease related problems.

Chronically ill persons are in most ways like other people. In addition, they must factor into their lives strategies for behaving normally in spite of moderate to severe limitations. To find out about the life of the chronically ill patient, the nurse need only invite conversation with the patient. What do you do during the week? How do you get out of your house? How do you manage to do the grocery shopping and laundry? Do you have friends? What kinds of things are you able to do with them? What kinds of problems does your illness cause in your daily activities? Working? Playing?

As staff get more data about their patients, they can understand their patients both as individuals and as a cohort of persons with particular needs growing out of their common medical problems. Nursing care should address these needs. For instance, patients with emphysema may need much more time for their morning care so that they can stop periodically to catch their breath. Ostomates may appreciate later scheduling for clinical studies so that they can follow their bowel regimens to completion in order to prevent accidents later in the day. Patients in the hospital might do better at tasks that take them from their rooms early in the day, before they tire and experience increased symptoms.

Last, the chronically ill person probably knows more about himself than his attending physician or nurses. He has preferences just like everyone else. This patient may exhibit some ritualistic behavior addressing health needs, and these should be regarded as time-honored strategies for feeling safe. Whenever possible they should be supported. The chronically ill patient needs to be a partner in his care. In truth, when this patient is discharged from inpatient care, he is usu-

ned over to himself. So hospital staff need to recognize re dealing daily with the patient's primary caregiver in the nity. This person is to be respected, taught when appropriate, hared with. The patient is also a teacher. He is a potential vol- e of data about suffering and coping. When appropriately asked, most patients are more than happy to share their knowledge.

REFERENCES

1. MAYO, L: *Problem and Challenge.* In: *Guides to Action on Chronic Illness.* National Health Council, New York, 1956.
2. STRAUSS, A AND GLASER, B: *Chronic Illness and the Quality of Life.* CV Mosby, St. Louis, 1975, pp. 7, 8.
3. Ibid., p. 143.

BIBLIOGRAPHY

ANGER, D: *The Psychological Stress of Chronic Renal Failure and Long-Term Hemodialysis.* Nursing Clinics of North America, September 1975, *10*, 449-460.

10
The Dying Patient

Lisa Robinson, R.N., Ph.D., F.A.A.N., C.S.

American culture places a high value on youth. Aging and dying are difficult to accept. Death itself, until recently, was not publicly discussed. It was a taboo topic, much as sex was in the last century. Thus, most individuals have not had an opportunity to develop an accepting attitude toward the dying process, and structures to help the individual work through his feelings have not been available.

In the past decade, however, with the impetus of research and publications by such leaders as Kubler-Ross, Cicely Saunders, and the Foundation for Thanatology, death has come to the forefront in people's awareness. Schools of nursing across the nation have developed courses on death and dying. Colleges, high schools, and even elementary schools offer programs to their students encouraging them to think and learn about death and dying. And still, the human being facing death has great needs.

The dying patient is beset with multitudinous problems. After he becomes aware of his condition, a complex set of emotions and defenses against anxiety are called into play to help the patient either to deny or ultimately to accept the prognosis. Kubler-Ross has done the definitive work on the stages of adaptation to dying.[1,2] She classifies these stages as denial, anger, bargaining, depression, and acceptance. All people do not go through all the stages. Some accept from the beginning. Others never accept. Still others end in resignation, a negative state of mind in which feelings about one's life and its meaning have not been worked through. The stages may be mixed, as when the individual experiences the stages of anger and bargaining simultaneously. There may be other combinations, or there may be fixations at one stage. In fact, the framework of these stages must be understood to be a rough guide in which the uniqueness of the individual is not overlooked. When a patient learns of his terminal prognosis, he may withdraw from contact with staff and friends. He experiences a stage of hopelessness. Some patients react by regarding their illness as something shameful—a punishment for bad deeds. Such is the case of a man who says to the nurse, ''What have I done to deserve this?'' Such regressive thinking is like that of a child who sees misfortune as a punishment for poor behavior. The nurse can recognize this regressive thinking and deal with the patient accordingly. Such a patient needs to be reassured that his illness is not a punishment. This is a beginning in helping the individual again experience himself as a person with worth.

Similar feelings were expressed by a young woman who had undergone a radical mastectomy when she queried the nurse, ''How can I face my friends? How are they going to treat me?'' Through her questions concerning the reactions of her friends, the careful listener would perceive that this patient was expressing some very negative feelings about herself. The patient anticipated isolation and rejection by her acquaintances because of her disease.

It is because of thoughts and feelings like these that patients retreat from other people. And all too frequently erstwhile friends abandon the dying because they are afraid and repulsed by evidence of their own mortality. Human interaction can be greatly decreased. This is the period when the patient seems uncooperative and unreachable. It is the initial phase of the psychological process of working through the knowledge of and feelings about one's own death. This state is identified by Kubler-Ross as denial, which is followed by anger. Some patients begin this process not with thoughts about ''How will others treat me?'' but with such thoughts as ''This can't be,'' ''This is a dream,'' or ''They've made a mistake. The laboratory has obviously mixed up their reports.''

The phases of denial and anger are difficult for the patient and are also difficult for the staff. The patient, not yet ready to move on with the process he must inevitably undergo, channels his energies into fighting himself, the staff, and others towards whom he displaces his anger. Yet this is a time when the patient needs an enormous amount of support. He is basically afraid because he perceives himself as alone in a situation that he cannot control. His perceptions are correct. He is alone; no one can die with him. He cannot control his dying; it will occur whether he wills it or not. The one monumental thing that the nurse has to offer is her presence and her willingness to be part of the patient's experience. To the extent that she can do so, she can alleviate his sense of aloneness. Yet this can be difficult because the patient includes those who are near and who offer potential support in his initial anger at the world and at death, which he cannot fight.

Not every nurse can tolerate being intimate with every dying patient. In any clinical area, however, there is usually someone who feels a potential for closeness with a given patient. When the individual is diagnosed as terminally ill, it is appropriate to explore with the staff which person will develop a close relationship with the patient. That is the person who makes a special effort to tolerate the patient's angry outbursts and his seemingly unappreciative behavior. This is the staff member who will respond with comments such as, "I can see how angry you are, and I wish I could help you get better." Or, "No. You're right. I'm not dying and I am glad of that, but I am also sad that you are, and I'm going to help you in every way that I can to be physically comfortable and not alone." Sometimes it is necessary to agree with the patient that his behavior is very difficult for his family and to point out that he has other options for dealing with his anger besides berating his relatives. Any of these types of statements are supportive as long as they are honest, deal with the problem straightforwardly, and indicate the staff's continued interest in the patient and their willingness to help in any way that is feasible.

When the patient has completed the struggles of the anger stage, he will then turn his focus inward, seem more depressed, and enter a period of grieving. His grief is determined by the quality of his interpersonal relationships, the use he makes of defenses such as denial, and the extent of his regression. If the patient has meaningful involvements with some people, as most of us do, he must anticipate the loss of these relationships. It is this impending separation that most patients fear, not death itself.

If the patient uses denial extensively he may not go through a period of grieving. This is because he has not faced the inevitability of separation. Regression serves to make the patient less cognizant of the value of his adult relationships. If the patient is severely regressed, he may entirely circumvent this period of grieving. Some patients become paranoid. They blame the world and the people in it for their fate. This is yet another means of trying to buffer the ego against an overwhelming realization.

During this grieving period, the patient will usually undertake a life review. At this time, he needs someone—family, friends, nurses, or chaplain—to listen as he thinks back over his life experiences, notes what he has accomplished or failed, and assigns meaning to his life. This is crucial in working through the process of preparation for death, and it should be encouraged by listening and asking questions if the patient's words need clarification.

If this phase is successfully traversed, the patient will move into the final phase of acceptance and he will no longer fight his impending death. The word *acceptance* is used here in the most flexible way. It is difficult to imagine any but the most religious or self-destructive person actually *accepting* death. The term as used here means that the patient is aware of his prognosis and is planning and preparing for it. Some preparation may be made through religious pursuits. Settlement of social and financial affairs is also necessary.

If these phases aren't successfully worked through, the patient will face death from a resigned position of anger and negativism. The patient who comes to accept his death is comfortable with it and has a basically positive attitude.

Denial is used by the patient who attempts to juggle time. He is aware that death is a necessary part of life, but he believes that his death will not occur in the near future. He polls those around him for corroboration. He compares his condition with that of patients with similar diagnoses and assures himself that he is not as ill as they. He blocks communication so that he cannot be alerted to his condition. Some patients coping by the use of denial become intensely active. They emphasize future orientation. By words and actions, they force family and friends to withdraw, so that patient and staff are forced into mutual isolation.

The patient who attempts to acknowledge his fate is not struggling with the idea of *death*. We cannot deal with something about which we have no information or experience. It is the *process* of dying that is thought about, fantasied about, and anticipated. The process of dying connotes decompensation, lingering debilitation, loneliness, emotional abandonment, and isolation from surviving friends and relatives. Dying means the ultimate loss of control over one's own life. This is the reason that some doomed people commit suicide. They take the opportunity to control the conditions of their last living experience, dying.

Caring for terminally ill patients is enormously taxing for the nurse. They experience personal and social losses when their patients die. If they are working on units where death is an uncommon event, such as obstetrics, then the psychological toll is higher. If the dying patient is a child, a young person, or one who has become well known to the nursing staff, his loss will be felt more keenly. This is understandable in philosophical as well as cultural terms. The nurse is then left with a legacy of grief.

The inner experiences of the nurse make her work with dying patients tremendously difficult. She must face, with each of her terminally ill patients, the fact that her own death is a facet of her life. She is forced to recognize her own mortality. She sees herself relinquishing life in the struggles of all her dying patients. This is the process of identification.

In addition to sadness and anxiety, nurses sometimes feel guilt. They respond unconsciously as though they have failed the dying patient in their role as caregivers. Sometimes nurses experience anger at the dying patient who does not respond to treatment. This is a reaction to frustration; the nurse wants to help the patient. She may also use denial. She unconsciously sets goals for a patient who will survive, not for her patient who is in reality dying. When the patient fails to respond to nursing intervention, the nurse is frustrated. She feels anger but cannot identify it. Nurses rarely are aware of the true character of these feelings. They only sense discomfort when they are near the object of their feelings, the dying patient.

Nursing education has not prepared the practitioner for verbal contact with dying patients. Emphasis has traditionally been on techniques, not on the process of dying. The nurse is rendered helpless when her task orientation cannot modify the patient's conditions. She has not been prepared to intervene meaningfully through verbal exchange.

All these factors engender extreme discomfort in the nurse. To work effectively and offer comfort and support to the moribund, the nurse has to become aware of her own feelings. She must be able to examine what she is doing so that her anxiety will not force her to withdraw from the situation. It is useful to the practicing nurse to become more fully aware of her thoughts and feelings about death and the dying patient. Attitudes that are conscious can be worked with and modified.

Often the situation is not a simple one in which staff and patient can communicate openly. If the doctor has chosen not to divulge information concerning his prognosis to the patient, the scope of communication is limited. The nurse is forced to become an actor in a drama not of her own choosing. She must focus on the future, which she knows is limited for this patient. Discussion of new symptoms and questions about prognosis are suppressed. This is a difficult situation. The nurse frequently resorts to the standard, "Ask your doctor." This is a poor response to the patient's query. It provides neither information nor support for the patient who is feeling anxious. The response communicates a rejection of the patient by the nurse, as well as a buck-passing attitude that places the nurse in a very unfortunate light. She is seen as grossly inadequate, rather than as a supportive, comforting, nurturing person that would be potentially helpful to the patient. This response also stifles communication. It tells the patient that there are acceptable and unacceptable topics for discussion.

If the nurse must defer to the attending physician, it is well if she can pick up some part of the patient's question for exploration. This may be accomplished by exploring with him his feelings about the topic or his expectations. Such a joint exploration might be instrumental in alleviating some of the patient's discomfort.

A particularly difficult situation presents itself when a patient who has not been told his prognosis is suspicious about it. The patient seeks information; he may test the staff in his attempts to ferret out the facts. One direct way of doing this is to ask various members of

the treatment team, "Am I dying?" If all answers are similarly negative, the patient is reassured that his case is not dire. However, he
may declare that he is dying to some member of the staff who is
uninformed about the patient's knowledge. The staff member, thinking that the patient has actually been told of his prognosis, might
confirm his suspicions by not questioning the patient's statement or
denying it.

The patient might also try to interpret the signs of his illness or
validate his suspicions by such means as new symptoms, tests, or
treatment, or by a move closer to the nurses' station. A change in
visiting regulations might provide evidence to the dying patient about
his condition.

In some instances it might appear that the patient really wants to
know the truth. This may well be, but the situation might also be one
in which the patient is trying desperately *not* to find out the truth.
This is a difficult problem for the patient. It is a complex operation of
"I know that you know and you know that I know that you know,
but *please don't tell me.*" The nurse is obliged by the physician's order
and the patient's wish to act out her role in the drama. The crucial
factor in the nursing care of the patient just described is to keep communications open. It is tempting to withdraw from him, but such a
maneuver means the realization of the patient's most basic fear—that
of separation and abandonment.

The psychological care of the dying patient is at least as important
as his physical care. In a case in which all hope has been abandoned
and the doctor indicates that the care of the patient will now focus on
making him comfortable, psychological considerations are of prime
importance.

Communication is the key issue. As the bridge between nurse and
patient, it prevents withdrawal and isolation. Communication with
the dying patient should allow him either to deny or to accept his
condition, as his emotional needs require. The nurse must not chide
the patient for not fighting to live. She must accept his impending
death. If the patient has accepted his fate, it is well for the nurse to be
a diligent listener and comforting companion. She may be instrumental in assisting the patient to preserve his identity and dignity as a
unique individual. It is imperative that the focus of the nurses' con-

tacts with the dying patient be on the here and now, rather than the future.

Mr. B. was a 30-year-old father of two girls, ages 2 and 4. He came to the hospital initially because of weight loss and pneumonia. While hospitalized, he was found to have leukemia. Mr. B. was placed on drug therapy which controlled his disease process well for almost two years. He was seen frequently in the outpatient clinics. Many of the staff nurses became familiar with this patient, owing to his frequent visits. He was regarded as a pleasant, intelligent, and sensitive person.

About two years after the original diagnosis was made, Mr. B. was admitted on the ward service. He had pneumonia. Mr. B. progressed satisfactorily during the first week of hospitalization. The doctors then decided to place Mr. B. on protective isolation. He was moved into a private room near the nurses' station.

When Mr. B. became morose, I was consulted. The patient had ceased talking and bantering with the staff, which had been the usual way that he related to those taking care of him. He remained pleasant, but the nurses saw that their patient had changed. The nurses described the situation: "Mr. B. knows he is going to die and he knows that we know, but he does not talk about it." When asked if they ever talked to him about his illness, the nurses said "Yes, but the discussions were in terms of the disease process rather than the person experiencing it."

Mr. B. was seen immediately. I introduced myself as a nurse who talked with patients facing difficult times and tried to help them. I told him I would try to assist him by sharing his experience in the hospital as much as possible.

The patient was seen daily for the next six weeks. He always took the initiative in the discussions. Sometimes the time was spent in conversation, sometimes in silence. The patient and I became well acquainted. There was little information provided about me, but my reactions to Mr. B.'s comments were expressed freely, in order that the patient could become aware of the nurse as a caring human being who was interested in him.

Mr. B.'s comments about his imminent death were not responded to factually but were interpreted as communications of feeling. When

he said "I am so worried," I responded, "It must make y
uncomfortable." Mr. B.'s feelings were elicited at frequer
order to allow him to be expressive, as well as to perm
that another person was aware of his feelings. This provided a ---
between the nurse and patient and combated isolation. It permitted
the patient to emerge as an individual.

As the interviews continued over several weeks, Mr. B. divulged
his intense worry about his wife and family. Social service and Mr.
B.'s priest were instrumental in alleviating some of these realistic worries. As resolution was found in this area, Mr. B. reverted to intro-
spection. The nurses were encouraged to visit this man frequently.
They were instructed to have as much physical contact with him as
seemed appropriate. This included touching him while conversing,
rubbing his back as part of morning and evening care, and feeding
him when he felt too weak to feed himself. This care was thought to
be strategic in communicating closeness and caring.

Mr. B. began to suffer from epistaxis and petechiae. He obviously
was alarmed about his new symptoms but did not verbalize this. The
daily visits were spent quietly. The patient and I, now well acquainted, seemed to have an awareness of one another's feelings. My
presence seemed to comfort him.

One day Mr. B. was transferred to the intensive care unit after an
extensive hemorrhage. He told me at this time that he was again
afraid. I communicated my understanding of his fear. On the fourth
day in the intensive care unit, I came to the area as breakfast was
being served. Mr. B. lay stretched out on his back, perspiring pro-
fusely. He was quite weak and spoke in whispers.

As I fed Mr. B. breakfast, he told me that he did not expect to live
much longer. I held his hand. Little was said during the visit, and I
promised to return in the afternoon. Mr. B. appeared resigned and
sad. He died quietly that afternoon.

The cardinal tenets of nursing terminally ill patients are these:
1. Be available and humane. *Make* time to spend with the patient. His
   opportunity for friendship and reciprocal communication is limited.
2. Allow the patient to set the pace. If the patient uses denial, do not
   try to break down this defense. Should an actual choice be neces-

sary, the patient's defensive operation must be supported. If the patient wishes to discuss his death, he should not be cajoled into changing the subject. This may comfort the listener, but it does not change the character of the patient's preoccupation.

3. Focus on the present. The future does not exist for the dying patient. Help him to cram all that is possible into today.
4. Keep communications open. When either patient or nurse feels that expression is no longer feasible, then the opportunity for supportive nursing care is lost. Within the confines of the attending physician's orders, every effort must be made to keep the channels of communication open.

REFERENCES

1. KUBLER-ROSS, E: *On Death and Dying.* Macmillan, New York, 1969.
2. KUBLER-ROSS, E: *Questions and Answers on Death and Dying.* Macmillan, New York, 1974.

BIBLIOGRAPHY

A way of dying. In SKIPPER, JK AND LEONARD, RC (EDS): *Social Interaction and Patient Care.* JB Lippincott, Philadelphia, 1965.

Death in the first person. Am J Nurs 70:336, 1970.

DUBREE, M, ET AL: *When hope dies—So might the patient.* Am J Nurs 80:2046, 1980.

GRIFFIN, J: *Family decision: A crucial factor in terminating life.* Am J Nurs 75(5):795, 1975.

GROUP FOR THE ADVANCEMENT OF PSYCHIATRY: *The Right to Die: Decision and Decision Makers.* Jason Aronson, New York, 1974.

GUNTHER, J: *Death Be Not Proud.* Harper Bros., New York, 1949.

HANLAN, AJ: *Notes of a dying professor.* Nurs Digest, 2:36, 1974.

HOLMES, M: *Nursing intervention with a dying patient.* In DUFFEY, M, ET AL (EDS): *Current Concepts in Clinical Nursing, Vol III.* CV Mosby, St. Louis, 1971, p. 37.

ILASCHENKO, J: *Assessment of anxiety and depression in the dying patient.* Topics in Clinical Nursing 1(2):39, 1981.

JACKSON, E: *Understanding Grief.* Abingdon Press, New York, 1969.

KRANT, M: *Dying and Dignity: The Meaning and Control of a Personal Death.* Charles C Thomas, Springfield, Ill, 1974.

KUBLER-ROSS, E: *On Death and Dying.* Macmillan, New York, 1969.

McNAIRN, N: *Helping patients who want to die at home.* Nurs '81 2(11):66, 1981.

NORRIS, C: *The nurse and the dying patient.* Am J Nurs 55:1214, 1955.

O'CONNELL, A: *When it's time to face dying*. Geriatric Nursing 2:273, 1981.

PARSELL, S AND TAGLIARENI, E: *Cancer patients help each other*. Am J Nurs 74(4):650, 1974.

PEARSON, L: *Death and Dying: Current Issues in the Treatment of the Dying Person*. Press of Case Western Reserve University, Cleveland, 1969.

RINEAR, E: *Helping the survivors of expected death*. Nurs '75 3:60, 1975.

SAUNDERS, C: *The last stages of life*. Am J Nurs 65:70, 1965.

SCHOENBERG, B, ET AL: *Loss and Grief: Psychological Management in Medical Practice*. Columbia University Press, New York, 1970.

SOBEL, D: *Death and dying*. Am J Nurs 74(1):98, 1974.

STORLIE, F: *The dying child*. Am J Nurs 74(6):1066, 1974.

VERWOERDT, A: *Communication with the Fatally Ill*. Charles C Thomas, Springfield, Ill, 1966.

11

The Problem Patient with Specific Personality Characteristics

Lisa Robinson, R.N., Ph.D., F.A.A.N., C.S.

Few people manifest characteristics of only one personality type. It is more common for the majority of us to demonstrate many traits derived from multiple ranges of personality characteristics. For the sake of simplicity and clarity, some trait clusters are described here. Any individual patient might exhibit several of the following behavioral patterns.

The anxious patient who worries constantly is not a stranger to the nurse. This is basically the kind of person who seizes upon the slightest upset and magnifies it into unrecognizable proportions. He seeks information from numerous sources and tends to misinterpret what he is told. He compares his condition and daily progress with that of the patients around him. It is likely that the results of the comparison frighten him.

This kind of patient will do better if he feels protected by competent, knowledgeable, strong caregivers. Discussion of the patient's illness should be limited to simple statements of fact. He should be given enough information to understand the basic problem, but not so much as to offer excessive material for conjecture or frightening fantasies. The nurse needs to be firm but kind. She must guard against involvement in the patient's anxious feelings. Her neutral, matter-of-fact interest in the patient can do much to stabilize him.

The patient who is uncomfortable accepting the nurse's attention may act very independent. This patient may go unnoticed in the daily routine because he takes care of himself and avoids nursing care. He may also be extremely critical of the efforts of those caring for him and may earn notoriety because of his verbose and negative critiques. He may attempt to instruct the staff in better patient management.

This patient does not easily discuss his own illness. His objectionable behavior is an attempt to avoid awareness of his basic fears regarding his safety. The nurse will find this patient less of a problem if he is made aware of the staff's approval of him as a strong person. If he is approached as a helping person and a possible source of aid, this type of patient will feel more comfortable. For instance, if this patient is prone to criticize the care of another patient, the nurse might actually solicit his ideas on improving the nursing care. This, of course, must be accomplished in a matter-of-fact manner. Any hint of derision or sarcasm would defeat the nurse's purpose.

Too often the overworked nurse finds herself struggling with a patient who is demanding and seemingly insatiable. He seems dedicated to the continuous scrutiny of himself and his illness. One gets the feeling that this patient is not so much concerned that something specific be done for him, as that things be done *constantly.* In other words, *quantity* seems to be the issue rather than *quality* of nursing care.

It is important to give this patient a sense of being cared for, indeed, of being appreciated. The nurse's humaneness, warmth, and caring are of prime importance. These qualities need to be communicated to the patient, and this can best be done by demonstrating a willingness to care for him.

If the patient's demands cannot be realistically met, the nursing staff must decide as a group what they can reasonably do. This establishes limits. The group must agree collectively that the limit is realistic. When there is group accord, there is likely to be consistency. The patient must be made aware of these limits in such a way that he does not feel chastened. The nurses should not experience guilt, because the limits they have established represent their objective evaluation of available time and resources. Guilt on the part of the nursing staff would be expressed as annoyance or anger directed at the patient. This would be detrimental to his well-being.

The patient is sometimes encountered who is extremely well organized and who adheres to a strict schedule. His day's activities are so ordered as to appear ritualistic. One gets the feeling that this person cannot be spontaneous in word or deed. The nurse will become aware of this patient's basic personality traits as she observes him. The patient may be rather precise in dress and conversation. His belongings are likely to be neatly arranged. Clothes, books, and toilet articles will show evidence of thoughtful selection and care.

This type of patient maintains his equilbrium by keeping himself and his environment under control. New and unexpected situations are not well tolerated. It is advisable to give this patient sufficient information about his treatment regimen and to prepare him for procedures before they are performed. The patient should be permitted as much leeway as possible in arranging his own activities. Wherever possible, the nurse should follow the patient's requests insofar as the scheduling and manner of carrying out daily activities are concerned.

The patient who impresses the nurses initially as a friendly, agreeable person sometimes becomes fairly aggressive in his pursuit of relationships with the staff. He is usually markedly articulate, and his tales and descriptions are colorful and often grossly exaggerated. This type of patient may be easily frightened. The hospitalization is difficult for him. This is seen when the patient becomes more flamboyant, hyperverbal, and overreactive.

When the patient is a woman, she may get into a competitive position, opposing the nurses. The latter are likely to develop negative feelings toward the patient. In an effort to gain approval and support from some quarter, this patient sometimes attempts to play off the nurses against the doctor. In a rather manipulative operation, the patient is likely to report that daily care is poor, the light is never answered, or the bedpan is not removed for some extended interval of time. (Of course one cannot justify this nursing care if the patient's reports are valid.)

In dealing with such a female patient, it is useful to help her feel comfortable about herself, about her appearance, her ability to attract and hold the nurse's attention, and her adequacy as a patient coping with an illness. This cannot be stated blatantly; however, the message is communicated by the nurse who comments, ''Your gown is awfully attractive,'' or ''I like that shade of lipstick,'' or perhaps, ''Could you teach me how to apply eye shadow like you do?'' Measures such as coming into the patient's room for a few minutes of unrequested conversation or dropping by to see if the patient wants anything are useful in getting the message to the patient that he or she is likeable. Such a maneuver will help to stem the patient's need to play off staff against one another.

Still another useful intervention is to allow the patient time to be with the attending physician alone. After chaperonage is provided during treatments or examinations, it is well to leave the patient and doctor alone, unless the latter specifies the contrary.

With patients of both sexes, a calm, matter-of-fact attitude is indicated. The nurse should guard against an intense involvement with the patient or overreacting to the situations that develop around him. Anxiety breeds anxiety. Should the nurse react to the patient's narratives with the same anxious feelings that motivated these dramatic accounts, patient and nurse can expect greater feelings of discomfort and few resolutions of the problems.

Information about the patient's illness and treatment should be given only after thought. The facts should be stated concisely and understandably. It is better to err to the side of brevity than to give superfluous information that might provide the basis for frightening speculations.

Some patients are perpetually on guard. They view others as potentially dangerous to their well-being. Hospitalization is an extremely distressing situation, because these patients are placed in a vulnerable position, and their normal vigilance is inadequate for buffering themselves against real and symbolic dangers. These patients' problems will be manifested by their behavior, which may be hypersensitive, suspicious, perhaps even querulous. They may remain aloof and unfriendly and behave in such a way that those around them think the patient regards himself as very important and powerful.

It is necessary to keep these patients informed about impending diagnostic studies or treatment or both. This is pertinent for allaying suspicions and helping the patients to prepare adequate defenses against new stresses. The staff should be courteous and friendly, but precautions should be taken that they do not appear aggressive in their pursuit of relationships with these patients.

The patient should set the pace during hospitalization. If he indicates a desire for friendship, then it is permissible to follow his lead. Should a preference for isolation be shown, it is well to respect this wish.

12

The Alcoholic Patient

Mary Ann Walsh Eells, Ed.D., R.N., C.N.

In the past, a diagnosis of alcoholism meant severe debilitation and early death. Modern treatment decreases this likelihood and helps the rehabilitated alcoholic to lead a full and productive life. Unfortunately, alcoholism still carries a social stigma in the American culture, which contributes heavily to treatment delays and a high level of denial of the illness. Vigorous and sustained efforts are made by both the patient and his family to avoid the diagnosis, so as to ward off the intense shame and guilt that it entails. This attitude constitutes a difficult (but not unmanageable) nursing problem in the hospital setting, since the nurse is usually in the position of dealing with an illness that the patient cannot admit he has.

The way in which the alcoholic patient is admitted to the hospital often augments his already high level of denial. If the multiple problems that accompany alcoholism should lead to hospitalization for psychiatric or physical illness, the alcoholic patient is convinced that this illness caused his drinking, not the reverse. His spouse, employer, or doctor may have given him an ultimatum that required him to enter treatment. If this life-saving act is accompanied by blame and moralizing directed toward the alcoholic, he resents hospitalization and views it as punishment. He thinks that "they" have caused the problem, not his drinking heavily. He may believe, for example, that his spouse's aggravating behavior causes him to drink, or that the unfair treatment at work at the hands of his supervisor or co-workers is the problem. He can be expected to hold to these views tenaciously.

His denial of any connection between his pathologic drinking and his hospitalization is automatic and unconscious.

The nurse can use one technique which, although unconventional, is very effective with alcoholic patients. His efforts to overcome whatever illness brought him to the hospital should be given a positive connotation.[1] Additionally, she should inquire about his drinking pattern, which will predictably elicit statements from him that he has no drinking problem. She should then take a position of agreeing with him—that probably he has no drinking problem. Interestingly, this position makes it possible for him to continue listening to her, instead of reacting immediately with denial. He feels appreciated as a human being, whose opinion is deserving of some respect. His receptiveness to her further comments facilitates instructing him about the progressive symptoms of alcoholism within the context of *if statements.* For example, *if* he had a problem, he would have a large capacity for alcohol and still be able to function. He would experience blackouts, or temporary amnesia, for events that occurred while drinking. Also, he would have problems at work and at home. The nurse can mention the usual expected physical effects, such as gastritis and hypertension, as well as the fact that he would begin to lose his ability to function sexually. His memory would not work as well as in the past, and he would have trouble judging spatial relationships, causing him to misjudge curbs or dent his car—that is, *if* he really is an alcoholic. Statements like these place the alcoholic patient in a peculiar position. The nurse has defused his usually oppositional reaction by agreeing with him initially, so that he is able to listen and learn. He may not act immediately upon the knowledge he is acquiring, yet the next time he experiences a symptom or event she has mentioned, he begins to make the connection with his illness. Often upon becoming abstinent, the patient will tell others about this nurse's effective approach and give her due credit for the influence it had upon his acceptance of treatment.

Another helpful strategy to use as an adjunct in this case is to comment directly upon the alcoholic patient's physical appearance, memory lapses, or other manifestations of his alcoholism. The alcoholic is unaware of how he objectively appears to others, even to the point of being oblivious to his reflection in a mirror. Left to his own devices, he readily dismisses even the most blatant signs of illness. Comments can be made about tremors, blood pressure elevations, spider angiomas appearing on his skin, gait disturbances, and other physical signs. He often will begin to realize that he is seriously ill—perhaps more so than the diagnosis of some other condition may indicate.

Secretly fearful that he may have a problem, he will often raise questions in the abstract about alcoholism in an effort to acquire information, as well as to clarify his confused thinking. The nurse should take advantage of the opportunity to inform the patient, especially about treatment resources. If the nurse herself has attended meetings of Alcoholics Anonymous as an observer, her personal description conveys a message of hope about the recovery of others. Similarly, if she is familiar with a variety of treatment resources—rehabilitation facilities, outpatient programs, and halfway houses—these become the patient's points of reference when he later becomes willing to submit to treatment.

When the alcoholic patient is admitted explicitly for treatment of his alcoholism, a somewhat different situation confronts the nurse. Mr. J., a 44-year-old successful salesman, was admitted to the alcoholism unit in a general community hospital. His twenty years of heavy drinking ended abruptly after a week-long drinking binge during a business trip to California. When he failed to return on a scheduled flight, his wife learned he had been detained by the police after jumping into his hotel pool fully clothed. Mr. J. had no recall of this event. Mr. J., an attractive, somewhat red-faced, but pleasant and engaging man, had been without alcohol for 48 hours. He received IV glucose and an antiemetic for his gastric upset and a mild tranquilizer that was to be discontinued the next day. His rest was fitful and he had mild hand tremors and considerable inner tremulousness.

Members of Mr. J.'s family seemed very subdued. An air of hopelessness prevailed. Although this was Mr. J.'s first hospitalization, his family seemed tired of the many inconvenient episodes due to his alcoholism. His two teenage daughters seemed uncaring and resentful toward their father. Mrs. J. had an air of worry and resignation. It was important to Mr. J.'s ultimate recovery to teach his family members about his illness and involve them in his care. The nurse chose to work with the most motivated family member, Mrs. J. The nurse also reflected Mrs. J.'s ambivalence in carefully chosen comments about the seriousness of the illness and how deeply it had affected the family, but reassured her that there was hope.

Families with an alcoholic member seldom know about the progressive organ damage that takes place, which includes a relentless and progressive atrophy of the brain, with associated cognitive and personality changes. Nor do they know that much of this damage is reversible but that recovery is prolonged, relapses common, and support systems for them absolutely necessary for months after abstinence is established.

Although Mr. J. experienced the gamut of central nervous system effects during his career of active pathologic drinking, he was frightened by the same effects when they occurred during hospitalization because he could not alleviate them by ingesting alcohol. His symptoms at hospital admission were chiefly dose dependent, a function of the amount of alcohol ingested, over what period of time, and the length of time that had elapsed since his last dose. This and other explanations that were given to him about his withdrawal from alcohol reduced his anxiety level and structured his otherwise chaotic, fear-provoking thoughts. The nurse explained to him also that he was seriously ill, but that he was no longer alone in battling his illness and that it could be put in the past. The disease aspects of alcoholism were communicated to the patient, especially their progressive but treatable and reversible nature.

This kind of information provides a coherent framework of explanation for the alcoholic patient. It usually does not occur to an alcoholic, as it did not to Mr. J., that he has been ill. The nurse explains that the physical and sometimes intense emotional symptoms he is now experiencing are an expected part of withdrawal from alcohol, but that they will end within a day or so.

The main central nervous system effect of alcoholism is autonomic hyperactivity, which accounted for Mr. J.'s anxiety, irritability, and gastric upset. His more-rapid-than-usual pulse and heartbeat and somewhat elevated body temperature were also expected effects. Mr. J. was told that he would probably experience a subjective sense of time passing by slowly; time might even seem to stand still. This was due to the paradoxical effect that occurs when the inner body processes speed up and, correspondingly, time in the external world seems to slow down. Mr. J. was told that he could also expect to have an acceleration of mental events—many things will pass through his mind—but that this too was to be expected during withdrawal. Should these autonomic nervous system symptoms speed up unduly, the nurse should be watchful for impending delirium tremens, usually experienced by no more than 5 percent of patients hospitalized for alcoholism,[2] and marked by considerable agitation, delusions, and usually vivid hallucinations. The nurse's interventions, which included helping to orient Mr. J. to reality by tracking events in logical sequence, were preventive.

Because of this altered perception of time, the patient should be assisted to maintain his grasp on reality by synchronizing his moment-to-moment experiences with the experiences of others in his environment. Even the simple exchange of impressions and ideas about everyday hospital events can help him to do so. As the nurse helps him to allocate experiences and events so that only a manageable proportion of them is handled immediately, his sense of self-control becomes better established.

Mr. J. required assistance from the nurse in getting beyond the immediate situation by transcending the present. Mr. J.'s childhood spiritual beliefs supported him at this point. He also had faith in the future when he was told that others had undergone what he was experiencing and they had gone on to live productive lives.

Most persons take for granted the three time frames of the past, the present, and the future, and automatically apportion their experiences to them, as appropriate. Actively promoting a livable time frame for the alcoholic patient is an essential, critical nursing intervention.

As Mr. J. emerged from the critical stages of withdrawal, the nurse helped him to anticipate similar events which might occur episodically during a *protracted withdrawal syndrome,*[3] which can last many months. These intermittent symptoms, persisting well into abstinence, are due to a slow resetting of the internal biological clock, which has become deranged by the effects of high blood alcohol levels upon the brain. Anticipatory control of the symptoms can be practiced during hospitalization, and this consisted chiefly of helping Mr.

J. pace himself and handling only immediate and necessary events. Other symptoms common during protracted withdrawal include fitful sleep and insomnia, often lasting many months, intense emotional peaks and valleys, and cognitive deficits, especially visuospatial and memory deficits.

Four days after his admission, Mr. J., detoxified from alcohol, was in great distress when the nurse entered his hospital room. Surrounded by his wife, his daughters, and his aging mother, Mr. J., a usually amiable man, looked humiliated and dejected. Mrs. J. was chattering on about all the odd jobs around the house that Mr. J. had neglected over the past two decades, that soon they would be able to buy a long-awaited new house, and that at long last he could be a real father to his daughters. His daughters were voicing their own expectations, most of which involved heavy expenditures related to upcoming college expenses. His mother stood silently by, witnessing the scene of demands and Mr. J.'s impotent response. As the demands became enumerated one by one, Mr. J.'s countenance became more dejected, as he added their expectations to his already long list of expectations, accumulated in his four days of abstinence. Under this kind of pressure, the nurse recognized that he might start drinking again, though some patients remarkably hold up under such pressures for some months before a relapse.

The alcoholic patient is always overwhelmed, once he realizes the full impact of his illness and its ramifications at every level of his life—physical, emotional, cognitive, social, and economic. Mr. J.'s thoughts over several days had touched upon every one of these aspects. He began to realize how ill he had been physically and that he was still not fully recovered. Emotionally, he was so labile that he began to wonder whether his emotions would ever again be under his control. Toward the end of his drinking, he had become aware of the cognitive losses—that he had been losing his grip on his job intellectually. The social and interpersonal losses seemed the most severe. His private thoughts often focused upon his wife's aggravating behavior, and he still partly believed this behavior had caused him to drink. He began to realize how much debt he had accumulated and how unproductive economically the past few years had been. He was in danger of losing his job, and probably would, he reasoned, given the unfair treatment he had received at the hands of his boss. Now, when he needed his family most he was chagrined to find that they were not supportive, only demanding. He concluded that it was all his fault. He was overcome by shame and embarrassment for his inadequate performance, particularly because it was witnessed by his children and his mother whom he should be taking care of in an adult fashion. He felt guilty for not having done so in the past.

Such realizations and emotions are not unusual for the alcoholic patient, once the alcohol is metabolically eliminated from his body. It is as if alcohol provided a protective cushion against all incoming stimuli from the environment, stimuli which could have helped him reach such realizations and take constructive, corrective action about problems. Without alcohol, Mr. J. felt denuded and exquisitely sensitive and vulnerable to all environmental stimuli. He was especially attuned to comments made by those particularly significant to him. Fortunately, most of the disorder and disorganization in his life was reversible, if he remained abstinent, and if he and his family could be patient about the process.

Mrs. J. was particularly important to the way in which the future would unfold. The nonalcoholic spouse is usually an overfunctioner[4] who fulfills virtually all of the role functions her alcoholic spouse does not. Mrs. J.'s response to her husband's hospitalization was anxiety laden, a dread of the unknown future with her husband sober. It was covered over by an exaggerated whistling-in-the-dark response and an exaggerated cheerfulness and hopefulness, filled with great plans for the future. At some deeper level, there was skepticism that her husband would actually stay sober this time, and sometimes this skepticism broke through in conscious thought. Mrs. J. would have to relinquish tasks which, though onerous, had contributed to her self worth. With Mr. J. sober, their relationship would change and intimacies would have to be renegotiated and perhaps re-established. Neither spouse felt up to these changes. Instead, their thoughts consisted of an ambiguous foreboding about the future. Mrs. J.'s anxious chattering and Mr. J.'s shame and dejection were their emotional responses to their fears of the future and their anticipated losses of the comfortable, though dysfunctional, patterns of their shared past. If one listened carefully to Mr. and Mrs. J., it became apparent that Mr.

J. was not alone in suffering some kind of warp in time. Mr. J. seemed overwhelmed mostly by his past, though somewhat worried about the future; Mrs. J.'s focus on time was an all-consuming view of the future and what would be accomplished, mostly by Mr. J.

In a busy community hospital, such as the one in which Mr. J. was hospitalized, various forces work against the recognition of, and interventions for, warped time frames of alcoholics and their family members, even though a balance and integration of past, present, and future time zones are essential to their recovery. Hospitals have their own time frames. There is the pressure of completing numerous tasks in a limited time; patients are observed for only small portions of the shift; and changing shifts of personnel and numerous observers make it difficult to establish whether patients are experiencing a continuity of time sequences during a hospital stay. However, the nursing staff were reporting growing concern about Mr. J. and the escalating difficulties he seemed to be having with his family. The family members had become bothersome to the staff also, particularly Mrs. J., who constantly queried them about Mr. J.'s discharge. She had become known on the unit as a troublemaker, and staff members began to attribute Mr. J.'s alcoholic drinking to his wife's obnoxiousness.

The nurse who had been caring for Mr. J. began to take part in some of the family visits, which by this time had deteriorated to Mrs. J. nagging her husband, the daughters chiming in, in agreement with their mother, and Mr. J.'s sullenness. Mr. J.'s mother was notably absent.

Certain patterns[5] were clearly evident in their communication with each other. The nurse noted that their interactions were markedly desynchronized. Mr. J. emphasized the past and his shame and guilt about his drinking; his wife focused upon her future expectations. It was obvious that the conflicting time frames also constituted conflicting values and expectations about behavior. Whereas Mr. J. was anxious to rectify the past by addressing it, Mrs. J. wanted to relegate the negative, drinking-related events to the past. Hers seemed the more healthy pattern. However, Mrs. J.'s expectations about the future were so impossible for Mr. J. to meet, they only inspired dread in him. The mismatch in time frames was also evidenced in the rate and rhythm of their speech patterns. Mrs. J. was overtalkative; Mr. J. exhibited a slow speech pattern which appeared to infuriate Mrs. J. who, in response, only talked faster. Their mismatched sequences were obviously at cross-purposes, but the incongruence in their verbal and nonverbal messages went unacknowledged by either of them. Most of what was said was unheard by the other and was left dangling.

After asking them whether they wished to communicate better with each other and gaining their permission with sheepish, embarrassed nods of assent, the nurse gave them the Circks test.* They were to think of the past, the present, and the future in the shape of circles, and draw circles to represent them.[6,7] Mr. J. drew a very large circle for the present and minuscule circles for the past and future. Mrs. J. drew the opposite—a very small circle for the present and large circles for the past and future. When asked to label each circle positively or negatively, Mr. J. labeled each of his three circles negatively. Mrs. J., on the other hand, labeled the past as very negative, the present as negative, and the future as positive. The nurse pointed out that each of them operated from a different time frame. In order to understand each other's point of view, each would have to listen to the other carefully. Pushing one's own point of view and time frame simply would not work; the other person's frame of reference was altogether different. It would be quite some time before Mr. and Mrs. J. would be able to negotiate their differences in this regard, and then only with the help of therapy after Mr. J.'s discharge from the hospital. But the nurse established an important reference point for them by showing graphically that assumptions could not be made about each other's thinking. Discussion and negotiation would have to take place in order for any progress to occur.

The nurse further reinforced these concepts by enlisting their cooperation in the construction of a family genogram,[4] a pictorial representation of both of their families that depicts their histories, generation by generation, from top to bottom on paper. It soon became evident

---

*Complete test instructions can be obtained by writing to the author at the University of Maryland School of Nursing, 655 West Lombard Street, Baltimore, Maryland 21201.

that Mr. J. could recall enough information to represent five generations of his family, though sketchily. But Mrs. J. had no information earlier than the generation of her parents. Even her parents' siblings were figures without names. The truly negative past reflected in Mrs. J.'s circles was also reflected in the limited information about her family's past. As they were asked about the geographic location of various family members, it became evident that both families were widely scattered. Family problems tended to be solved by geographic moves, cutting off the past and moving toward an unknown future, which often ended disappointingly. Mr. and Mrs. J. had faithfully followed this familial pattern with many job changes and uprooting geographic moves. Their sense of historical continuity had been lost.

As the family history was gathered, a sufficiently negative past in the lives of their respective families became established, so as to instigate a powerful motivation for change for Mr. and Mrs. J. It is human nature to tend toward the status quo, until it is demonstrated that unmanageable disorder and disintegration have occurred. In itself, this is a powerful force for change. If it can be shown that such disorder has existed for generations, all the better. This seems to move the current generation to improve their lot for themselves and their children. Alcoholism had existed in the families of Mr. and Mrs. J. for as many generations as they could recall. They were genuinely concerned about perpetuating the pattern and the legacy they would leave behind them. It became apparent to them that they had been stuck in time for years, with an incapacity to move forward and progress. The drinking problem that had been the cause of Mr. J.'s hospitalization became a shared family problem, out of which emerged a sense of shared purpose. They became determined to break a vicious cycle of transmission from generation to generation.

It would be remiss to leave unmentioned the progressions and regressions of the J. family after Mr. J.'s discharge from the hospital and over a period of several years. The nursing staff heard that Mr. J. did attend meetings of Alcoholics Anonymous, which were held on the hospital grounds. The family therapist who saw the J. family on an outpatient basis once commented that they were overcoming their problems. Mr. J. has never been readmitted to this community hospital for the treatment of alcoholism, although he did stop by once to mention that, for the first time in several generations, both sides of the family are free from alcoholism.

REFERENCES

1. WATZLAWICK, P, ET AL: *Change*. Springer, New York, 1974.
2. AMERICAN PSYCHIATRIC ASSOCIATION: *Diagnostic and Statistical Manual of Mental Disorders*, ed 3. American Psychiatric Association, Washington, D.C., 1980.
3. EELLS, MAW: *Principles of treatment for the alcohol abusing client and family*. In CRITCHELY, D AND MAURIN, J (EDS): *The Psychiatric Mental Health Clinical Specialist: Theory, Research and Practice*. John Wiley & Sons, New York (in press).
4. BOWEN, M: *Family Therapy in Clinical Practice*. Jason Aronson, New York, 1978.
5. MELGES, FT: *Time and Inner Future*. John Wiley & Sons, New York, 1982.
6. COTTLE, TJ: *The circles test*. J Proj Techniques Personality Adjustment 31:58, 1969.
7. EELLS, MAW: *Timekeeper spouses who contribute to equilibrium states in alcoholic family systems*. In TRONCALE, L (ED): *A General Survey of Systems Methodology. Vol 2: Applications to Real Systems*. Society for General Systems Research, Louisville, KY, 1982.

BIBLIOGRAPHY

ESTES, NJ AND HEINEMANN, ME (EDS): *Alcoholism: Development, Consequences and Interventions*, ed 2. CV Mosby, St. Louis, 1982.
THUNE, CE: *Alcoholism and the archetypal past*. J Stud Alcohol 38(1):75, 1977.

13
The Geriatric Patient with Cognitive Dysfunction

Kenneth Solomon, M.D.

Disorientation, a frequent clinical problem of the elderly, involves various aspects of cognitive dysfunction. Contrary to common belief, however, cognitive dysfunction in the elderly is not a problem that is seen with the frequency of other psychiatric dysfunctions, especially depression, alcoholism, and chemical dependency.[1] Cognitive dysfunction, regardless of cause, affects only 6.2 percent of the population at the age of 65,[2] with a gradual increase in incidence to 20 percent at age 85. In the general hospital, older patients seem to have a much higher incidence of disorientation for several reasons: They are likely to have chronic physical problems that cause cognitive dysfunction, and the elderly are more likely than younger persons to develop physical illnesses. The various causes of cognitive dysfunction (which will be described below) account for more than one fourth of all admissions of the elderly to psychiatric hospitals other than public psychiatric hospitals.[3]

Senility is an umbrella term for cognitive dysfunction in the elderly that should never be used. Related to it is that commonly observed syndrome called sundowner's disease. Neither term describes an actual medical diagnosis. Cognitive dysfunctions in the elderly have a physical cause. The loss of orientation with resultant aberrant behavior and fright that is observed in some institutionalized elderly patients after dark has an underlying physical cause. It is functionally destructive to relate these problems to that myth called senility, which is usually assumed to be inevitable and untreatable. In *approximately one fourth of patients, this underlying cause or disease is treatable, and treatment will lead to complete or partial reversibility of the cognitive dysfunction.* For those whose underlying causes cannot be altered, nursing care may be effective in arresting the course of the disease. Supportive psychosocial interventions may lead to alteration in the elderly patient's disorientation.

Elderly patients may appear disoriented when they are admitted to the general hospital, or they may become so after undergoing diagnostic tests or therapy. The latter group of patients tend to do better than patients who have been disoriented for longer periods of time, because the patient who suddenly appears disoriented may be evaluated and treated rapidly and effectively. The chronically disoriented patient may have a long-standing or irreversible condition.

Cognitive dysfunctions, with disorientation being the commonest symptom, should be viewed as instances of brain failure. Brain failure can be described along four dimensions: symptoms, course of acute onset, etiology, and prognosis (Fig. 1). It has been taught that cognitive deficits can be categorized as acute reversible brain syndromes and chronic irreversible brain syndromes. This conceptualization suffers from oversimplicity, for there are endless combinations of the four dimensions with resultant variations in the outlook for effective treatment of the patient's symptoms. These symptoms range from pure delirium to pure dementia. These conditions look alike (Tables 1

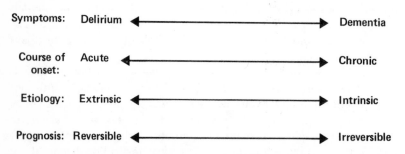

FIGURE 1. Dimensions of brain failure.

TABLE 1 Primary Symptoms of Brain Failure

1. Memory loss
2. Disorientation
3. Apraxias
4. Agnosias
5. Aphasias
6. Loss of problem-solving skills
7. Impulsivity
8. Disturbance of sleep cycle
9. Weight loss and generalized debility
10. Cortical release phenomena
11. Alterations of level of consciousness

and 2),[4] although pure delirium is characterized primarily by changes in the *level of consciousness,* with deficits of attention and secondary memory deficits.

Ms. J., a 62-year-old widow, was admitted for a cerebral arteriogram following an episode of transient loss of awareness. She was alert and cooperative on admission. During her workup and preparation for the test she was friendly toward the nurses and helpful. Fol-

TABLE 2 Secondary Symptoms of Brain Failure

1. Exaggeration of premorbid personality characteristics
2. Anxiety
3. Depression
4. Delusions
5. Hallucinations
6. Confabulation
7. Catastrophic reactions
8. Inability to perform activities of daily living
9. Social consequences

lowing the arteriogram, Ms. J. was unable to sit up for several days. She slept constantly, unless aroused, ate minimally, and spoke only when shaken awake and requested to respond. When the nurses tried to engage her in conversation Ms. J. reported that she "felt drowsy" and could not remember why she was in the hospital nor what had happened to her since her admission.

Sometimes changes in the level of consciousness may not be obvious, especially if the patient is hyperalert, rather than drowsy or seemingly dull (obtunded).

In pure dementia, there is a normal level of consciousness, and the deficits of memory are primary. Thus, in delirium the change in the level of consciousness is the primary symptom; in dementia, the primary symptom is a memory deficit. In reality, most patients experience a variety of both delirious and dementing symptoms.

Some patients become disoriented suddenly, such as following a cerebrovascular accident (CVA), while others may seem to slip away insidiously, such as those with Alzheimer's disease. Some elderly individuals have subchronic cognitive deficits resulting from malnourishment or silent hematomas. In these hard economic times, it is not unusual to hear about destitute persons starving, mixing hot water and ketsup to make soup, or eating cat food. Even for the elderly who are not financially pressed, living alone often leads to irregular meals that are of dubious nutritional quality. Depression, shrunken gums upon which dentures no longer fit, or a decreased ability to digest may cause the elderly to make do with one can of soup per day or some tea and crackers. Old persons tend also to be frail and unsteady. Orthopedic and/or neurological problems, such as parkinsonism, may cause the individual to lose his balance easily and fall. If the head strikes a corner table, or chair, or even the floor, subdural hematomas may result. Symptoms of brain failure may be extrinsic following head trauma; intrinsic, as in the case of multiple small clots that alter the blood supply to the brain; or a combination of both extrinsic and intrinsic factors. The clinical course may be completely or partially reversible, irreversible and stable, or irreversible and progressive.

The symptoms of cognitive dysfunction can be considered in two groups. The first, or primary, symptoms can be directly traced to the underlying neurological dysfunctions.[5] Secondary symptoms arise from the elderly person's attempts to cope with his deficit and also from the struggles that he has with others who share the patient's efforts to cope. Primary symptoms of cognitive dysfunction are listed in Table 1. The main symptom is memory loss, which usually follows a predictable pattern. Essentially, recent memory is lost first, followed by remote memory. Memories that are charged with feeling are retained longer than those that are neutral. Memories of whole events, or gestalts, are retained longer than memories of specific details.

Mr. L. is a 65-year-old retired widower. He lives alone in an apartment and stubbornly refuses assistance from his children, neighbors, or family. He frequently leaves his apartment and forgets why he left and is seen wandering aimlessly around the streets. Mr. L.'s greatest pleasure is going to baseball games. His sister picks him up each evening in the summer and drives him to the stadium. There, they sit together in the sister's box and watch the game. Mr. L. always knows who he is and who his sister is, but when other family members join them in the box, he frequently does not recognize them but hides his disorientation through harmless banter and superficial chatter.

Disorientation is frequently a symptom that is first observed in the patient who has brain failure. The process of disorientation is always sequential, that is, it begins as disorientation to time, then to place, then to present situation, and finally, in severe disease states, to self. The memory deficit and disorientation may first be noticed by a sense of vagueness as the person talks to the nurse, doctor, or family. Events and memories will not be fleshed out, giving the listener a vague picture of the patient's views. This state of affairs occurs before the patient exhibits frank memory deficits or disorientation.

Other neurological symptoms may appear, such as the inability to perform complex motor acts (apraxias). In early cognitive deficits this is often erroneously viewed as willful refusal, depression, or laziness, and may include difficulties with using eating utensils, tying shoelaces, or buttoning clothes. It may also include such commonly seen behavior as putting clothes on backwards.

Another set of of neurological symptoms includes the inability to recognize items or people in the environment (agnosias). This problem is particularly distressing to family members. For them it is an abyss that cannot be bridged. The loving dad or mom who always made pancakes on Sunday morning or took the gang to little league baseball is gone. In that person's place is a look-alike, a stranger; someone who *should* know but doesn't. The family member with this deficit is surely alive, but he is functionally dead. The shared life between patient and family is over.

Another neurological symptom is aphasia, or the inability to speak. Early aphasias are usually a nominative aphasia, in which the person has difficulty finding names for objects in his environment. The progression of this symptom causes the expansion of the inability to communicate. Gradually the person becomes less able to take in communication, as well as to speak. This is called a mixed receptive and expressive aphasia. The elderly person has difficulty understanding abstract language and undergoes a gradual simplification of thought processes. This process may underlie concrete responses to the request to interpret proverbs that is part of the mental status exam, a typical example being, "What does it mean that 'people who live in glass houses should not throw stones'?" "It means that they may break the house." The elderly individual with this neurological process cannot think abstractly so that he does not comprehend that the glass house is a *symbol* of one's own vulnerabilities. For the patient, the word house connotes a structure in which one lives. Likewise such a patient when asked "What would you do if you found a stamped addressed envelope on the ground?" would likely answer, "I would open it." The patient's judgment has been altered by his contracted capacity to think. In this constricted state thinking no longer expands to consider issues of ethics and morality.

Loss of impulse control is another primary symptom. It may lead to an increased show of affect in response to either internal or external stimuli. In the extreme such a response is termed a catastrophic reaction. Catastrophic reactions may be evident by sudden and what seems to be unprovoked crying, or verbal or physical outbursts of anger. When not provoked by external stimuli or the environment, it is usually provoked by the person's internal psychological state. This will be discussed later.

There may be changes in the patient's level of consciousness. A diminished level, often seen as either semicomatose or dulled, is easily recognized as evidence of brain failure. More difficult to assess is a change of consciousness in the direction of a *hyperalert* state. A hyperalert state is frequently associated with paranoid thinking in which the patient fears that forces are out to hurt him in some way. A diminished need for sleep and diminished purposeful motor activity are often the first signs of a delirious hyperalert state. The attention span may also be altered, which may be partly related to memory deficit.

Secondary symptoms occur in approximately 95 percent of patients with Alzheimer's disease[6-8] and are very common in other patients with cognitive deficits. Secondary symptoms (see Table 2) are often related to coping strategies used by the elderly for dealing with stress (Fig. 2). While the challenge of stress is common to all age groups, from the elderly it exacts a high price. The older individual experiences a diminished sense of mastery over his internal and external environment. Stressors for the elderly include a variety of unpredictable and sudden losses, including losses in the individual's social support system, loss of social roles, and a variety of other losses[1,8-12] (Table 3). In addition, the elderly must cope with the stress imposed by daily victimization in four dimensions of their lives: physical, economic, attitudinal, and role.[1,9-13] For persons with impaired brain function, memory deficits, sudden and severe physical illness, removal from one's usual surroundings to a hospital, and meeting a variety of new people are in themselves stressors that may provoke a realistic sense of loss of mastery.

When an elderly person is stressed by the loss of mastery, other issues also emerge. Feelings of helplessness are compounded by the

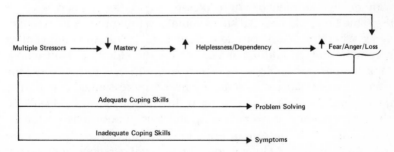

FIGURE 2. Stress and coping in the elderly.

TABLE 3 Losses of the Elderly

I. Loss of social support system
   1. Spouse
   2. Siblings
   3. Friends
   4. Parents
   5. Children
   6. Other kin
   7. Neighbors
II. Loss of social role
   1. Occupational role
   2. Shift to tenuous and informal roles
   3. Gender role
III. Miscellaneous losses
   1. Health
   2. Independence
   3. Income
   4. Mobility
   5. Adequate housing
   6. Leisure activities

need to depend on others while not wanting to do so. This is complicated in the hospital because the patient wishes to adopt the sick role with its attendant feelings of helplessness and dependency, while at the same time, the hospital staff promotes a rapid return to independence when the acute episode is resolving.[14-17] This apparent conflict may represent an additional stressor for the elderly person whose coping repertoire is already overextended. To add to his woes, the patient may be labeled as senile by health professionals who do not understand the patient's behavior or the reasons for it.[16-19] Helplessness, dependency, powerlessness, and loss impose tolls on the elderly patient that he cannot hope to overcome. These traumas are compounded through interaction with hospital personnel who do not understand the plight of the elderly and who react by labeling and censuring.

The elderly individual without brain failure or cognitive deficit is hard pressed to cope with these stresses. For the patient who has a cognitive deficit, the job is Herculean. This patient may not be able to use previously learned coping skills, because they are not remembered or because the new situation is not recognized as similar to one in which the person coped successfully in the past. Left without coping strategies, the elderly person may react to stress with physiologic changes,[20] irrational behaviors, exaggerated feelings, or a combination of reactions that can be viewed as catastrophic. Behaviors and underlying feelings will be related. Indeed, the type of behavior observed will be associated with the intensity of the underlying feeling (Fig. 3).

Behavior problems are more likely to occur in persons who are overdependent or pseudo-autonomous or those who regress when stressed. Patients who experience sadness or even depression will manifest less anxiety with increased psychomotor retardation. The person who has been egocentric or one who has somaticized problems during the majority of his life is likely to cope with stress through these means again.

All patients who show cognitive deficits must be medically and psychiatrically evaluated to rule out any treatable causes of brain disease[21] (Table 4). Additionally, the patient's family needs evaluation in order to assess the patient's and the family's capacity to cope and to plan supportive and psychotherapeutic interventions. A thorough

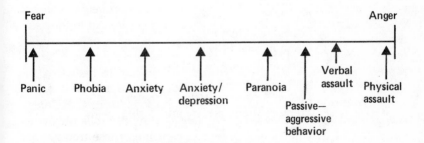

FIGURE 3. Psychopathologic symptoms in the elderly and their place on the fear/anger continuum.

TABLE 4 The Psychogeriatric Evaluation

1. History of the present episode
2. Past and present medical history
3. Drug history
4. Past psychiatric history
5. Psychosocial history
6. Review of systems
7. Physical exam
8. Neurological exam
9. Mental status exam
10. Laboratory exam

history is vitally important and in it should be a careful description of all drugs taken by the patient, for drugs may cause cognitive deficits.[22] A psychosocial history (Table 5) and mental status examination[23-26] (Table 6) round out the picture of the patient.

TABLE 5 Psychosocial History

1. Family history
2. Developmental history
3. Educational history
4. Occupational history
5. Current financial situation
6. Current housing
7. Past and present leisure time use
8. Premorbid personality and coping skills
9. Current psychosocial stresses
10. Current psychosocial resources

TABLE 6 Mental Status Examination

1. Appearance
2. Level of consciousness
3. Attention
4. Mood
5. Affect
6. Activity level
7. Thought process
8. Thought content
9. Perception
10. Memory
11. Intelligence and abstraction
12. Orientation
13. Judgment
14. Insight

As can be seen in Table 7, just about every disease described in standard textbooks of internal medicine can cause transitory or permanent cognitive dysfunctions.[27] However, there are certain diseases that are much more likely than others to cause reversible or irreversible brain failure. One of the most common causes of reversible cognitive deficits is depression. The depressed individual usually demonstrates an increase in concrete thinking, difficulty with attention span, mild memory deficits, a lack of energy and will to answer many questions, and poor personal hygiene.[28] Occasionally, the severely depressed older patient may demonstrate urinary or bowel incontinence[29]; thus the older depressed patient may easily be confused with the patient with organic impairment. To complicate matters, many medications and medical conditions may also cause depressive symptoms. Furthermore, the individual with a mild cognitive deficit may respond to it by becoming depressed.

All drugs, over-the-counter or prescription, licit or illicit, may cause cognitive deficits.[22] Psychotropic drugs, alcohol, antihypertensive medications, cardiovascular medications, cimetidine, and hormones

TABLE 7 Causes of Reversible Brain Failure

1. Depression
2. Drugs (prescription, over-the-counter, illicit, alcohol)
3. Nutritional (especially hypovitaminoses)
4. Intracranial mass lesions (especially sequelae of head trauma)
5. Metabolic (especially dehydration, hypoglycemia)
6. Endocrine (especially thyroid, adrenocortical, pituitary)
7. Vascular
8. Cardiac
9. Fever and infections
10. Hepatic
11. Pulmonary
12. Extracranial malignancy
13. Renal

are common offenders.[22,27] Drug toxicity may exist in the presence of therapeutic or even less-than-therapeutic blood levels of these drugs. Since the elderly are frequently overmedicated, cognitive deficits are often easily treated by removal of all medications that are not necessary for life-threatening disorders. As mentioned before malnutrition and sequelae of head trauma may also cause reversible brain failure.[30]

The most common cause of irreversible brain failure is Alzheimer's disease.[31] Multiple small strokes (multiple infarct dementia) are the next most common cause. The third most common cause of irreversible brain failure is a combination of Alzheimer's disease and multiple infarct dementia. Finally, untreated reversible causes of brain failure may eventually lead to permanent damage.

Unfortunately health care providers are often satisfied to label the elderly patient as senile so that an adequate evaluation is not made.[32-37] Personnel respond to the patient's weaknesses rather than assessing his remaining strengths and supporting them. Nurses need to explore their own thoughts, feelings, and biases about the elderly in order to have a clearer idea about the interventions that can be brought to bear on problems faced by the elderly in the health care system.[36-38]

Following an assessment, appropriate intervention is implemented if further cognitive dysfunction is to be halted or current deficits reversed. Appropriate supportive intervention may obviate the need for psychotropic medication in the majority of patients. It is important for the health care provider to understand the elderly patient's actual problem and his capacity to master that problem. Equally significant is the patient's perception when coping has proven insufficient.

In some cases, psychotropic drugs may be used for specific problems such as psychotic symptoms or frequent catastrophic reactions[1,38-39] (Table 8) or severe depression (Table 9). In many instances supportive nursing measures will alter the problem. One useful strategy is for the nurse to *coach* the patient in appropriate and effective coping strategies (see Fig. 2). In such an instance it is imperative that the health care provider understand what is age- and capacity-appropriate for the elderly patient. Acute anxiety in the elderly is not changed by the use of medications[40-41] but may be modified by teaching breathing exercises based on the Lamaze childbirth method.[42] Relaxation exercises from stress management models are also useful.[43,44] The nurse describes and actually *models* these movements for the patient and then helps the latter to develop them. Agitation may be reduced by walking with the patient or giving him specific tasks to do. For example, patients may wheel other patients in wheelchairs, hand out food trays, or empty wastepaper baskets, under supervision, as ways of channeling their energy and giving them a sense of purpose. Helplessness, dependency, and powerlessness secondary to multiple forms of loss have been identified as major stressors for the elderly. The experience of being *needed* is therapeutic. It is important, however, for the nurse not only to seek the patient's help but to communicate that the help is truly needed and appreciated. Busy work is demeaning. Communicating the nurse's regard for the elderly patient and the nurse's appreciation of assistance removes the aura of busy work from these tasks. Occupational therapy and activities therapy can also be used to channel the energy that, if unchanneled, leads to agitation. Behavior modification paradigms may also be helpful with other behavioral symptoms.[44,45]

TABLE 8 Antipsychotic Drugs

I. Phenothiazines
   A. Aliphatic
      1. Chlorpromazine (Thorazine)
      2. Promazine (Sparine)
      3. Triflupromazine (Vesprin)
   B. Piperidine
      1. Thioridazine (Mellaril)
      2. Mesoridazine (Serentil)
      3. Piperacetazine (Quide)
   C. Piperazine
      1. Prochlorperazine (Compazine)
      2. Trifluoperazine (Stelazine)
      3. Butaperazine (Repoise)
      4. Perphenazine (Trilafon)
      5. Fluphenazine (Prolixin, Permitil)
      6. Acetophenazine (Tindal)
II. Thioxanthines
      1. Chlorprothixene (Taractan)
      2. Thiothixene (Navane)
III. Butyrophenones
      1. Haloperidol (Haldol)
IV. Dihydroindolones
      1. Molindone (Moban, Lidone)
V. Dibenzoxazepines
      1. Loxapine (Loxitane, Daxolin)

Modification of behavior is one broad strategy for intervention; the other is modification of feelings. The latter is usually accomplished through desensitization, channeling of the feeling into action, or simple expression. Many individuals, especially men (even those without cognitive deficits), have difficulty identifying their feelings.[12] They often experience only a vague discomfort. People with cognitive deficits may also misidentify, mislabel, or somaticize uncomfortable feelings

TABLE 9 Antidepressant Drugs

I. Tricyclics
   A. Iminobenzyls
      1. Imipramine (Tofranil, Presamine, Imavate, Janimine, W.D.D., SK–Pramine)
      2. Trimipramine (Surmontil)
      3. Desipramine (Norpramin, Pertofrane)
   B. Dibenzoheptadienes
      1. Amitriptyline (Elavil, Endep)
      2. Nortriptyline (Aventyl, Pamelor)
      3. Protriptyline (Vivactil)
   C. Dibenzoxepins
      1. Doxepin (Sinequan, Adapin)
   D. Dibenzoxazepines
      1. Amoxapine (Asendin)
II. Tetracyclics
      1. Maprotiline (Ludiomil)
      2. Trazodone (Desyrel)
III. Monoamine Oxidase Inhibitors
      1. Isocarboxazid (Marplan)
      2. Tranylcypromine (Parnate)
      3. Phenelzine (Nardil)

that arise from stress. Nursing intervention to modify this experience includes helping to draw out the patient's feelings and giving the patient permission for these feelings to be verbalized. It is useful for the nurse to talk about anger, fear, and sadness and to initiate discussions about feelings and the usefulness of sharing one's feelings with another. Encouraging the patient to share his feelings occurs by asking simple questions about the patient's experience to lead him into the desired subject.

Helplessness can be minimized by requiring the patient to function as autonomously as possible. This is accomplished by assigning specific behavioral tasks to the patient and minimizing the sick role as much as the patient's physical condition will allow. The latter item may prove more difficult for the staff than the patient, because the hospital is geared to role reciprocity: The object of nursing care, the patient, is expected to get in bed, be compliant, and passively accept the staff's ministrations. However, as noted previously, the sick role leads to helplessness and further psychopathology in the elderly.[7,16,17] To counter this process, the patient should wear street clothes as much as possible, stay out of bed, and perform as many tasks of daily living as possible.

An increased sense of mastery is achieved by creating opportunities for the patient to succeed. Various projects in occupational therapy and activities therapy that can be completed by the elderly patient allow him to see concrete results of expended efforts. Mastery is increased by insuring that the elderly patient maintains a choice in and autonomy over his environment. Choices of clothing, food, and activities in which the patient wishes to be occupied should all remain with the patient. More complicated choices also should be the patient's, as much as is appropriate. Two responsibilities of nursing are to help the patient create options so that choice exists and to act in a way that conveys to the patient that he, and not the nursing staff, is responsible for the patient's behavior.

An important part of both the prevention and management of secondary symptoms is the reduction of stressors acting on the patient. The guidelines in *The 36 Hour Day*[46] are valuable for nursing. Adequate nutrition and regular exercise are essential.

For delirious patients, multiple nursing measures may reduce symptoms. These measures include one-to-one care in a room with dim lights and soft music. A modicum of sensory stimulation avoids both sensory *deprivation* (and its resulting psychotic symptomatology and agitation)[47] and sensory *overload* (also with secondary agitation). A blaring television or radio may do more harm than quiet music or one-to-one nursing care and light conversation. Correction of hearing and visual deficits will often modify paranoid symptoms better than antipsychotic medications. The patient should remain out of bed as much as possible, not only to prevent the development of decubiti, but more important, to increase the amount of tactile and visual stimulation. Touch, if it is accepted by the patient, should also be used as much as possible as a form of communication and sensory stimulation.

When communicating with a patient who is cognitively impaired, the nurse should use very simple, clear, and concrete language, at a level that the patient understands. (It is important to ascertain what the patient understands and not to make assumptions about the patient's ability to understand; it is as easy to talk *above* the patient's head as it is to talk down to the patient.) Whenever possible, the nurse should be at the eye level of the patient, even if it requires the nurse to sit or kneel. The patient should be looked at face to face and spoken to slowly. Loud volume is frequently unnecessary, even in the patient with moderate hearing deficit, because it distorts the voice and makes it difficult for the patient to understand what is being said; it is also often perceived by the patient as patronizing.

Procedures should be explained to the patient several times prior to their performance. Each step of the procedure should be explained and all questions answered. For instance, when taking blood pressure the nurse might say: "Mr. Jones, I am going to take your blood pressure. I am going to roll up your sleeve. Now I am going to put this cuff around your arm. I am going to fill up the cuff to put pressure on your arm; this may be a little uncomfortable." Frequent verbal and written reminders of activities of daily living are also necessary if the patient is to maintain autonomy. Although it is easier and faster for a nurse to dress the patient, being allowed to dress himself is advantageous to the patient's mental health and functioning. Reminders and instructions on tasks should be as simple as possible. Complex behaviors must be broken down into more simple ones. For example, a request to get dressed may be too complex for many patients with cognitive deficits. Instructions to put on each item of clothing may be necessary.

Reality orientation[49] can also be beneficial. Formal reality orientation classes allow the patient some social interaction and structured activity during the day. But reality orientation is a twenty-four-hours-a-day, seven-days-a-week job. The patient should always be in rooms with windows, so that he can tell whether it is day or night and so that he can identify the season and the weather. Whenever entering a patient's room (after knocking, of course), one should always introduce oneself and remind the patient where he is. Frequent reminders of time, place, and current events should occur during general conversation. Important personal items from home, such as photographs of family members, his own clothing, and his own blanket, pillow, books, and towels increase the patient's ties to present reality. Visiting hours should generally be unrestricted so that familiar individuals can help the patient retain a hold on reality.

SUMMARY

It has been noted that nurses, like members of society in general, stereotype the older individual as a physically and mentally deteriorating, helpless individual. It is important to realize that even the older patient with cognitive dysfunction and brain disease has a functioning brain that is capable of and wants to learn and to respond to human love, warmth, and contact.

REFERENCES

1. SOLOMON, K: *The elderly patient.* In SPITTELL, JR, JR (ED): *Clinical Medicine. Vol XII.* In BRODY, EB (ED): *Psychiatry.* Harper & Row, Hagerstown, MD, 1981, pp. 1-14.
2. KAY, DWK: *The epidemiology and identification of brain deficit in the elderly.* In EISDORFER, C AND FREIDEL, RO (ED): *Cognitive and Emotional Disturbance in the Elderly.* Year Book Medical Publishers, Chicago, 1977, pp. 11-26.
3. REDICK, RW, KRAMER, M, AND TAUBE, CA: *Epidemiology of mental illness and utilization of psychiatric facilities among older persons.* In BUSSE, EW AND PFEIFFER, E (EDS): *Mental Illness in Later Life.* American Psychiatric Association, Washington, D.C. 1973, pp. 199-231.
4. AMERICAN PSYCHIATRIC ASSOCIATION: *Diagnostic and Statistical Manual of Mental Disorders,* ed 3. American Psychiatric Association, Washington, D.C., 1980.
5. WELLS, CE: *The symptoms and behavioral manifestations of dementia.* In WELLS, CE (ED): *Dementia.* FA Davis, Philadelphia, 1971, pp. 1-11.
6. GOLDFARB, AI: *Clinical perspectives.* In SIMON, A AND EPSTEIN, LJ, (EDS): *Aging in Modern Society. Psychiatric Research Report No 23.* American Psychiatric Association, Washington, D.C., 1968, pp. 170-178.
7. GOLDFARB, AI: *Minor maladjustments of the aged.* In ARIETI, S AND BRODY, EB (EDS): *American Handbook of Psychiatry, Vol III,* ed 2. Basic Books, New York, 1974, pp. 820-860.

8. SOLOMON, K: *Alzheimer's disease: The subjective experience of the patient.* Geriatric Consultant 1:22, 1982.

9. SOLOMON, K: *The depressed patient: Social antecendents of psychopathologic changes in the elderly.* J Am Geriatr Soc 29:14, 1981.

10. SOLOMON, K: *Personality disorders in the elderly.* In LION, JR (ED): *Personality Disorders: Diagnosis and Management,* ed 2. Wiliams & Wilkins, Baltimore, 1981, pp. 310–338.

11. SOLOMON, K AND HURWITZ R: *Stress, coping, and the older gay man.* Presented at the 59th Annual Meeting of the American Orthopsychiatric Association, San Francisco, CA, Apr 2, 1982.

12. SOLOMON, K: *The older man.* In SOLOMON, K AND LEVY, NB (EDS): *Men in Transition: Theory and Therapy.* Plenum Press, New York, 1982, pp. 205–240.

13. SOLOMON, K: *Victimization by health professionals and the psychologic response of the elderly.* In KOSBERG, JI (ED): The Abuse and Maltreatment of the Elderly. John Wright-PSG, Littleton, MA, 1983, pp. 150–171.

14. PARSONS, T: *The Social System.* Free Press, New York, 1951, pp. 428–473.

15. WILSON, RN: *The Sociology of Health: An Introduction.* Random House, New York, 1970, pp. 13–32.

16. SOLOMON, K: *Social antecedents of learned helplessness of the elderly in the health care setting.* In LEWIS, EP, ET AL (EDS): *Sociological Research Symposium Proceddings (IX).* Commonwealth University, Richmond, 1979, pp. 188–192.

17. SOLOMON, K: *Social antecedents of learned helplessness in the health care setting.* Gerontologist 22:282, 1982.

18. SOLOMON, K AND VICKERS, R: *Attitudes of health workers toward old people.* J Am Geriatr Soc 27:186, 1979.

19. NYE, I: *Is choice and exchange theory the key?* J Marriage Fam 40:219, 1978.

20. SELYE, H: *The Physiology and Pathology of Exposure to Stress.* Montreal, Acta, 1950.

21. SOLOMON, K: *Assessment and intervention in psycho-social dysfunction in the aged.* In JACKSON, OL (ED): *Clinics in Physical Therapy. Vol 6. Geriatrics.* Churchill Livingstone, New York, 1983, pp. 84–112.

22. LEVENSON, AJ: *Neuropsychiatric Side-Effects of Drugs in the Elderly.* Raven Press, New York, 1979.

23. MENNINGER, KA: *A Manual for Psychiatric Case Study,* ed 2. Grune & Stratton, New York, 1962.

24. STEVENSON, I AND SHEPPE, WM, JR: *The psychiatric examination.* In ARIETI, S (ED): *American Handbook of Psychiatry, Vol I,* ed 2. Basic Books, New York, 1974, pp. 1157-1180.

25. MACKINNON, RA: *Psychiatric history and mental status examination.* In KAPLAN, HI, FREEDMAN, AM, AND SADOCK, BJ (EDS): *Comprehensive Text book of Psychiatry, Vol I,* ed 3. Williams & Wilkins, Baltimore, 1980, pp. 906–920.

26. FOLSTEIN, MD, FOLSTEIN, SE, AND MCHUGH, PR: *Mini-mental state: A practical method for grading the cognitive state of patients for the clinician.* J Psychiatr Res 12:189, 1975.

27. LIBOW, LS: *Pseudo-senility: Acute and reversible organic brain syndromes.* J Am Geriatr Soc 21:112, 1973.

28. BECK, AT: *The Diagnosis and Management of Depression.* University of Pennsylvania Press, Philadelphia, 1973.

29. BLAZER, DG II: *Depression in Late Life.* CV Mosby, St. Louis, 1982.

30. FOLLIS, RH, JR: *Pellagra.* In HARRISON, TR ET AL (EDS): *Principles of Internal Medicine.* McGraw-Hill, New York, 1966, pp. 374–378.

31. ROTH, M: *The natural history of mental disorders arising in the senium.* J Ment Sci 101:281, 1955.

32. MCGUINESS, AF AND KNOX, SF: *Attitudes to psychogeriatric nursing.* Nurs Times 64 (Suppl):127, 1968.

33. KAYSER, JS AND MINNINGERODE, FA: *Increasing nursing students' interest in working with aged patients.* Nurs Res 24:23, 1975.

34. ROBB, SS: *Attitudes and intentions of baccalaureate nursing students toward the elderly.* Nurs Res 28:43, 1979.

35. DYE, CA: *Attitude change among professionals. Implications for gerontological nursing.* J Gerontol Nurs 5:31, 1979.

36. SOLOMON, K AND VICKERS, R: *Stereotyping the elderly: Changing the attitudes of clinicians.* Presented at the 33rd Annual Meeting of the Gerontological Society of America, San Diego, CA, Nov 25, 1980.

37. SOLOMON, K AND VICKERS, R: *Stereotyping the elderly: Further research on changing the attitudes of clinicians.* Presented at the 34th Annual Meeting of the Gerontological Society of America and 10th Annual Meeting of the Canadian Association on Gerontology, Toronto, Ont, Nov 10, 1981.

39. SOLOMON, K: *Haloperidol and the geriatric patient.* In AYD, FJ, JR (ED): *Haloperidol Update: 1958–1980.* Ayd Medical Communications, Baltimore, 1980, pp. 155–173.

40. SOLOMON, K: *Benzodiazepines and neurotic anxiety. Critique.* NY State J Med 76:2156, 1976.

41. SOLOMON, K AND HART, R: *Pitfalls and prospects in clinical research on antianxiety drugs: Benzodiazepines and placebo—A research review.* J Clin Psychiatr 39:823, 1978.

42. BING, E: *Practical Lessons for an Easier Childbirth.* Bantam, New York, 1969, pp. 36-52.

43. JACOBSON, E: *Progressive Relaxation.* University of Chicago Press, Chicago, 1938.

44. WOLPE, J: *The Practice of Behavior Therapy.* Pergamon Press, New York, 1969.

45. SHAEFER, HH AND MARTIN, PL: *Behavioral Therapy.* McGraw-Hill, New York, 1969.

46. MACE, NL AND RABINS, PV: *The 36 Hour Day: A Family Guide to Caring for Persons with Alzheimer's Disease, Related Dementing Illnesses, and Memory Loss in Later Life.* Johns Hopkins University Press, Baltimore, 1981.

47. SOLOMON, P: *Sensory Deprivation.* Harvard University Press, Cambridge, 1961.

48. MARX, HL: *Hear Again Live Again.* Beltone Electronics Corporation, Chicago, p. 14.

49. STEPHENS, L: *Reality Orientation: A Technique to Rehabilitate Elderly and Brain Damaged Patients with a Moderate to Severe Degree of Disorientation.* American Psychiatric Association, Washington, D.C., 1969.

14
The Special Patient

Lisa Robinson, R.N., Ph.D., F.A.A.N., C.S

What characterizes anyone or anything as special? It can be said that an object is special because it stands out from similar objects. The same can be said for the special patient. This is the hospitalized person who looks or acts or is treated differently from other patients. Sometimes the difference is good; sometimes it is bad.

The special patient may be different because of a physical attribute such as the disease for which he is being treated; because the patient is a very important person (VIP); or because he may cause people in the hospital system to act differently, that is, cause role instability among the staff. For example, after an attempted assassination, President Ronald Reagan held special patient status when he was admitted to a large teaching hospital in Washington, D.C., for treatment of his punctured lung. One can only imagine what occurred in the emergency room that was suddenly filled with people, in the operating room to which he was hastily wheeled, and in the recovery room to which he was taken after his surgery. A documentary on television 12 months after the event gave some clues as to the many scenes that transpired during the President's hospitalization. Personal communication with involved staff corroborated my expectations that the hospital ran very differently.

Sometimes the cause of deviation in a hospital's procedures is not a special person but an unusual condition.

Mr. W., a 40-year-old salesman, was admitted with a provisional diagnosis of tetanus. He appeared toxic and in pain upon admission.

Staff were warned that this patient could decline rapidly. He was treated with massive doses of toxoid as well as antibiotics. In spite of these measures, the patient became sicker and convulsed intermittently. By this time, most of the personnel in the hospital had heard about the unusual patient and many of them dropped by the room to get a glimpse of the patient-celebrity.

The pace of visiting staff increased as the patient's condition declined. Convulsions were now approaching the frequency of status epilepticus. Any noise or even the whisper of a breeze seemed sufficient to trigger the next seizure. The patient's room resembled a Disney set as every article in it that could vibrate was wrapped in Kerlex to decrease its potential noise. Even the door jamb was padded. Medication did not stop the convulsions. Staff were in constant attendance with oxygen, curare, and other supportive measures. It was all to no avail, however, and the patient died.

Mrs. L. was admitted to a large teaching hospital for removal of a tumor resting on her spinal column. It was determined that the tumor, which had rendered the woman paralyzed, had involved the cord itself. The surgical staff, determined to help their patient, elected to try a new innovative procedure: They designed a prosthetic spinal column to insert after the removal of a portion of her own diseased one. Special procedures and instruments were produced to complete the complicated surgery. The patient, informed about the risks of her surgery, knew that she would remain paralyzed after it, but that if she recovered, she would at least be able to sit up. Also, the procedure seemed to be her only hope for survival from the tumor. Needless to say, this patient became the darling of the Department of Orthopedics and the celebrity of the hospital at large, and her progress was followed intermittently by local television stations. By the end of the first month of hospitalization, Mrs. L. was becoming increasingly demanding towards the Chief of Orthopedics, her surgeon. He, in turn, was increasingly irate with the nurses and residents caring for his patient. The patient did not progress as well as had been hoped and it was not only the hospital family who knew about her trials and tribulations, but also anyone with a television set was apprised of her problems. As Mrs. L. slowly recuperated, she regressed, becoming childish and petulant. She felt slighted by some, while she enjoyed the excessive attentions of others. She bargained with the doctors for extra privileges and reported those who she felt denied her. Finally, after many months of convalescence she was discharged and went home in a specially outfitted van. The staff breathed many sighs of relief. Owing to an ascending infection, Mrs. L. was soon readmitted, amidst the hoopla of radio and TV coverage. She struggled to survive, as each day's report was beamed into the homes of thousands. Her eventual death was mourned by many.

Another group of special patients are persons who have the potential to use their power to cause the health care system to operate differently from normal. The group includes such persons as actors or other performers, philanthropists, wealthy people, and those with ties to other important people or to persons recognized as significant in the health care system. Such a patient was admitted to the trauma center. He was a staff aide to a government official. He was badly hurt in a car accident. While hospitalized, many government officials came to the unit to visit this patient and his condition was monitored by local government officials and by the media. The unit to which he was admitted was also funded from state resources. Thus, the staff of the unit experienced additional stress when administering to this special accident victim.

The roles of hospital staff are clearly defined and executed as long as the patient assumes patienthood, facilitating an ongoing reciprocity of roles with health care providers. Problems arise when the patient does not act appropriately. Main[1] writes that the course of hospitalization for such a patient is marked by loss of objectivity on the part of the therapeutic team with whom the patient forms intense, exclusive, and mutually *harmful* relationships. In such cases, when the patient is admitted, he seeks special considerations such as different visiting policies, leaves of absence, or unusual requests. The attending physician may also seek special care for his patient. There may be a history of failure on the part of the patient to improve, but with "*this* regimen" (prescribed by a sensitive and intelligent clinician), the patient will recover. Staff compete to respond to the patient. The patient forms special ties with selected staff and soon the staff are split. The physician may no longer be recognized as the head of the team. Some nursing staff may be unwilling to act from medical directives, because they believe that they understand the beleaguered patient better than the rest of the team. In fact, this may be the case; however, the situation is sufficiently common that it is likely not to be the case.

In the classic situation, staff members who are favored by the patient are isolated from the rest of the staff. The patient and specially designated staff are likely to regard hospital policies as "insensitive, unfeeling, harsh and inadequate" for the patient's "subtle and poignant needs."[2] The patient who has asked repeatedly for special attention and favors asks those of staff who have abetted him to also join him in a mutual examination of medical orders and hospital rules. In their quest to secure special treatment, staff and patient conduct complicated cross-checks with various other staff members in order to find "loopholes."[3] Eventually the ploys wear thin. Staff who have become involved re-examine their own roles and become aware of their uncertainty as caregivers and members of a working team. In their growing anxiety, they question "Am I a bad nurse (doctor)?" Rescue fantasies give way to bitterness toward the patient, and staff's attention shifts from the patient to themselves. They may perceive that the patient's relationships are destructive because they are intense, short-lived, and almost always disappointing. The patient had had magical expectations of care. Staff have tried to meet them, stretching themselves unrealistically and failing. The goals that were once so obvious and the objectives that were originally routine are found to be ineffective. Before the process can be halted, the self-confidence of the staff gives way to self-doubt. Blame, irrational accusation, and guilt erode normal professional relationships. Slippage of roles is noted as staff struggle to regain equilibrium in a morass of discontent. This process leads to withdrawal from the patient.

M.L. is a 16-year-old girl who was admitted to a medical ward because of a pre-leukemic condition. She has had this blood disorder for five years. She is treated with supportive measures and blood transfusions whenever admitted and is usually discharged with moderate improvement in her condition. On this hospitalization she has created havoc on the unit with her behavior. M.L. refuses to wash and feed herself, claiming that she is too weak. She succeeds in getting various nurses to do these activities of daily living for her. Several days ago she refused to get out of bed; when the nurse insisted, the patient acquiesced and then stooled on the floor. The house officer in charge of the case refuses to help the nurses by supporting their appropriate care plan calling for consistent limit setting. The doctor says if the girl wants to be fed and bathed she should be.

The VIP often receives special patient status. This individual has personal influence or professional status and can exert unusual pressure upon staff. Typically, he is influential. The patient's power may stem from a highly placed government job, such as a senator or mayor of the city, or from fame as a performing artist, or the patient may be a physician, or even the private patient of an influential doctor. Sometimes the patient picks up the bedside phone and calls directly to the hospital administrator when he wants something. Special privileges are assumed, and normal operating procedures on the unit may be suspended without particular forethought and decision-making. Often the patient's admission results in temporary upward delegation of authority within the hospital hierarchy to create special conditions for this politically sensitive person.

The son of the chief of surgery was admitted for biopsy of a suspicious lump in his groin. Subsequently, it was found that the 19-year-old boy had a testicular cancer. The attending surgeon, the patient's family, and shortly the entire hospital staff were grieving the youth's condition. Either the boy's father or the attending physician was constantly on the phone to the nursing supervisor or the front office seeking one thing or another. The attending surgeon had written an order that no one was to speak to the boy about his diagnosis. Nursing students caring for him noted that he frequently asked them questions about his condition. They felt that their hands were tied. When the surgeon was apprised of this, he wrote another order prohibiting his patient from being cared for by nursing students.

Mr. C.R., a 66-year-old industrialist, was admitted to the C.C.U after suffering a myocardial infarction. His condition stabilized after three days, and he began demanding to be sent to a private room. He hated the monitors and the lack of privacy. Mr. C.R. was obviously used to giving rather than following orders. The nurses and physicians alike grew quickly frustrated from his constant demands, and they were soon willing to discharge him to a private room with nurses around the clock. While hospitalized he set up a veritable bunker in his large and commodious room. Several phones were installed as well as a conference table for groups that came to consult with Mr. C.R. Mr. C.R. did not like the hospital food (he said it was unpalatable), so his meals were brought in by local caterers. Staff did not often visit this patient. The attending physician made rounds once a day. The head nurse stuck her head in the room once in the morning to offer a perfunctory hello. The floor nurses said that they saw no reason to enter this patient's room, because he was "covered with specials." When the patient's nurses went out of the room for meals, they always told the floor staff they were leaving, but several times Mr. C.R. put on his light to no avail.

In most cases of VIP embroilments, staff esteem decreases. This leads to their withdrawal from the patient. The patient usually escalates his demands. Staff experience guilt as a result of their intense anger at the patient (or family or physician who support the patient's demands). Sometimes staff deny the severity of the patient's illness in an effort to distance themselves from him. Their anger increases as the VIP patient appeals to the powerful figures in the administrative hierarchy, demonstrating his lack of trust in the immediate care providers.

The management of the special patient focuses on prevention rather than cure. Once the process is underway, people are hurt. No one wins. The patient does not have his needs met, staff feel inadequate, and administrators are vexed and bewildered. It is imperative that the potential for problems be recognized before the process is set in motion. Signs of impending disaster are fervent requests from the attending physician or administrators for special consideration of the patient. This is sometimes coupled with comments about one staff member's special sensitivity or professional competence. When the patient presents a history of frequent change of health care providers without clear-cut reasons, this is yet another clue that trouble may be in the offing. The patient and his family may be openly critical of past care. Frequent calls and requests to administration for information may be observed. Frequently the ward staff are surprised to be last to hear about some change in the patient's care or a deviation in policy regarding this patient's hospitalization. At the same time it may be noted that supportive services called in to see the patient leave scant notes on the chart. The patient himself may be noncompliant. The most common situation (and most malignant) is the split that occurs among staff between the ones who believe that they understand the patient and want to help and those who do not like the patient and withdraw from him and who even feel antipathy toward the righteous but misled group. This is a late phase of the special patient syndrome and is to be avoided if possible.

It is most important that staff not let communications break down among themselves. They need to discuss openly their feelings about the patient. It is necessary to examine *issues* about the patient, which are separate from the feelings that staff experience about the patient and about each other. Any shift from usual hospital policies and routines should be first discussed in the group before being enacted. Communications with administration should also be kept open and used to share problems. Administration should be alerted to strategies that will be used to maintain this patient in his appropriate role in the system. Control should be kept at the staff level while at the same time maintaining flexibility in the patient's behalf, as long as it results in good patient care. This means that the staff must not be seduced into an inflexible, reactive position to the patient's bids for special favor and control; rather, staff should hear the patient's comments, requests, and actual needs and evaluate each on its separate merit. Rules and procedures should be followed unless there are extremely compelling reasons not to. In that case, the larger work group must make final decisions about deviation. Limits must be sensitively applied and the patient's pathological behavior controlled. As structure returns to the system, staff morale increases and role instability will disappear.

REFERENCES

1. MAIN, TF: *The ailment.* Br J Med Psychol V(30): 129, 1957.
2. POLLACK, I AND BATTLE, W: *Studies of the special patient.* Arch Gen Psychiatry 9:344, 1963.
3. Ibid.

BIBLIOGRAPHY

KILLILIA, M: *Karen.* Prentice-Hall, Englewood Cliffs, NJ, 1962.

MASSIE, K AND MASSIE, S: *Journey.* Knopf, New York, 1975.

MAUKSCH, H: *The nurse: Coordinator of patient care.* In SKIPPER, J AND LEONARD, R (EDS): *Social Interaction and Patient Care.* JB Lippincott, Philadelphia, 1965.

POOLE, V: *Thursday's Child.* Fawcett, New York, 1980.

WEINTRAUB, W: *The VIP syndrome: A clinical study in hospital psychiatry.* J Nerv Ment Dis 138(2):181, 1964.

15

The Health Care Provider As Patient*

Lisa Robinson, R.N., Ph.D., F.A.A.N., C.S.

A member of the hospital "family" was admitted under urgent conditions. On the evening prior to admission, the patient had experienced sudden loss of vision in one eye. A visit to the patient's doctor in the morning confirmed that the symptoms reflected neurological deficits of a serious nature. In the subsequent series of events, the patient saw consultants who confirmed earlier findings and the patient was admitted to the hospital.

The patient came to the unit late in the afternoon. She was unescorted and without luggage. External appearances led us to believe this person, who was casually dressed, was in good spirits and actually a bit ebullient. The patient complied with the admission procedure willingly, indicating her familiarity with it. When questioned about the reason for her admission, she stated quite casually the nature of the neurological deficit. (It was reported later by the admitting nurse that she wondered about the inappropriateness of the patient's affect at that time.) The patient's spouse, who was also of the hospital family, arrived during the admission procedure. The admitting nurse noted that both individuals displayed a seemingly happy, carefree attitude. The remainder of day one was uneventful.

Day two began with a series of tests, including electroencephalogram, chest and skull x-rays, electrocardiogram, brain scan, and lumbar puncture. The lumbar puncture was performed by a member of the patient's family. It was noted that during this procedure the patient displayed the talkative, cheerful demeanor of the previous day. Orders were received that day to administer ACTH 40 U in 500 cc D/W every day for 10 days. When the 10 bottles of fluids were placed in the patient's room she said very brightly and with a big smile, "Well, I guess I'll be here for 10 days anyway."

The patient had many visitors during the ensuing days. Many were medical colleagues. The patient asked and received numerous answers to her many questions concerning the outcomes of the diagnostic studies, differential diagnoses under consideration, probabilities of exacerbations, probable locations of neurological lesions, and so on. The answers came from all levels of hospital personnel—attending physicians through house officers.

My interest in this case was engendered after the initial workup and initiation of steroid therapy. I noticed that the patient followed a rigid schedule of activities. The morning began quite early (6:30 to 7:00 A.M.) with a trip to the utility room to get on the scale. Smiles and good mornings were accorded any and all persons met in transit. This was followed by careful, almost meticulous preparation for the day, via selection of bedwear and morning care. By the time breakfast arrived, the patient seemed ready to "hold court." The I.V. was usually begun by 9 A.M. and the patient remained in bed until 3 P.M. when the therapy was discontinued. After this, she arose, met with any remaining visitors, had dinner, and then began the evening ritual of a bath and hairwash. When not talking on the phone, the patient was usually found reading. The books in the room appeared to be of a technical nature and related to her work. This, then, provides a description of a seemingly good patient who happened to be one of the hospital family. Although the staff did not recognize it, she was also a patient who did not receive the type of care usually given in cases such as hers.

I soon discovered another world in which this patient functioned beyond that one in which we interacted. My first glimpse of this nightmarish other world occurred when I was told that before leaving the shower room each evening, the patient turned out the light before opening the door and experienced the subsequent sensory deprivation in an effort to become familiar with blindness, that is, "to try it out." She admitted at this time to looking out the shower room window, many stories above the street, and watching the people come and go from the hospital. She felt that these people were far removed—essentially in another sphere of time. As far as I can correlate, it was during this period that the attending doctors were undecided on a final diagnosis but were sharing with the patient each new finding and its possible implications. The patient did not ask for, nor share with the nursing staff, any information of a clinical nature. Because of her position as a member of the medical community, the nursing staff did not attempt to evaluate this patient's feelings about her experience nor did they initiate plans to support her.

Shortly after I heard about the preoccupations of the shower room, the patient confided in me that she often thought of suicide. The idea seemed to be prompted by the sight of the windows in the bedroom and the shower room. (It is important to recall that the patient occupied a room high above the street.) She reported debating the issue of living or dying because the current pressures on her were so overwhelming, and, projecting beyond this hospitalization, the future appeared particularly grim in terms of progressive debilitation and repeated hospitalizations. She said that suicide was only one of several means she considered for coping with the newly discovered problem. (This patient was reported to be a highly active person both physically and mentally.)

Shortly after this, she described an awareness of approach and avoidance movements in the behavior of others. She compared her perceived field to the sighting device of a rifle or a radar screen. The patient at the center of the field felt able to plot the movements of others closer and farther away from her. This sensation was not accompanied by sadness or joy; it was merely accepted. At a later date, the patient described feelings of loneliness as the avoidance behavior of others became evident. At this time, too, she expressed awareness that the nursing staff had distanced themselves, with the exception of two individuals who maintained close, meaningful contact. The patient did not attempt to communicate these feelings of loneliness and unrest to the other nurses. During the course of these psychological events, the patient also reported the onset of chills and tachycardia every day at about 8:30 A.M. She was psychiatrically sophisticated and reasoned that the response was psychologically stimulated by one of two events: either the arrival of the I.V. nurse or that of one of the consulting physicians who visited regularly at this time and shared much clinical information.

Towards the end of the hospitalization, the patient told me that she was no longer preoccupied with thoughts of suicide. These thoughts had been of some magnitude. We can understand this because the patient reported great fear of heights but said such considerations were secondary to the knowledge that death would be swift and final. But now the continuation of life seemed of first priority; the reason—a family, still young, had to be raised. The patient's degree of infirmity was still not great enough to override the priority of the children's needs.

The patient was discharged; final diagnosis was undetermined. According to the attending physician, the diagnosis would have to be confirmed by time, perhaps 5 to 10 years. The patient planned to convalesce as prescribed and then return to a waiting hospital post.

The important considerations of this case are several. Communications between nursing staff and attending physicians were minimal. Had the nursing staff known what information the patient had been given, they could have been aware of the patient's potential problems and might have had the opportunity to help her as she tried desperately to cope with the overwhelming amounts of frightening information presented.

The ritualistic behavior of this patient had significance, and its observation by the nursing staff could have been used in a therapeutic manner. In retrospect, we know that the patient was highly anxious. Had we not been seduced by her title and identity, we might have used our observations of ritualism as a symptom of efforts to fend off the loss of identity that this patient was apparently experiencing under the pressure of her progressing neurological symptoms and the quantities of incomplete information concerning diagnosis and prognosis.

The nursing staff failed for this patient. She might have received the psychological support she needed had staff been able to recognize the tremendously complex and catastrophic issues being weighed; however, they could not glimpse the patient's inner world, eclipsed as it was by her special patient identity. Had the nurses identified this medical person's struggle, they might have recognized her need to receive information in amounts small enough to cope with. They might have supported this patient's defenses, that is, suppression and denial, in order to hold back the ultimate knowledge until the patient's mind was prepared to receive the facts and to place them in a realistic framework.

Because the patient is a doctor or nurse does not mean that he really wants to treat himself or be a part of the committee that treats him. At base, we are all human beings aware of our existence. We deny real knowledge of our finiteness, in most cases, until we are faced with evidence of this condition. It is frightening to face such an awareness suddenly.

It is at this point that a medical background becomes less relevant. Finiteness is crucial. The human mind can tolerate only so much bombardment without help in sorting out the threads of the meaning of life and the end of life, the meaning of being and of nonbeing. Though the patient with a medical background might question the results of his tests, it is well to try to evaluate how much information he really wants and can handle. Such a process requires sitting with the patient, permitting him to talk, responding in a manner that demonstrates our similar human qualities, and showing, if possible, that we are trying to understand the patient's world. If the patient indicates that his "circuits are overloaded," all those involved in the patient's care should be made aware of it.

The nurse must be alert to the special needs of the health care provider who is a patient, because these individuals may be more vulnerable to unintentionally poor care. Nurses and others on the health team should be vigilant in their investigation of the patient's real needs and the planning and implementation of care for him.

BIBLIOGRAPHY

MAIN, T: *The ailment.* Br J Med Psychol 30:129, 1957.

POLLACK, I AND BATTLE, M: *Studies of the special patient.* Paper read at the Maryland Association of Private Practicing Psychiatrists and the Maryland Psychiatric Society, March 14, 1963.

ROBINSON, L: *The medical person as a patient.* Am J Nurs 71:1728, 1971.

WEINTRAUB, W: *The VIP syndrome.* J Nerv Ment Dis 138:181, 1964.

16
The Role of the Nurse

Lisa Robinson, R.N., Ph.D., F.A.A.N., C.S.

The nurse is responsible for her patient's welfare, both physical and psychological. She medicates him, administers treatment, and tries to create an environment in which he can come closest to a state of psychic equilibrium. The nurse becomes an advocate of the patient. She speaks to him of the factors influencing his condition, both those emanating from him and those impinging upon him. She explains to the patient those things being brought to bear upon his illness by the medical team, and she interprets to the team the thoughts and feelings of the patient that he might be unable to communicate himself and that have some bearing on his course of treatment.

The nurse must cope with many factors as she attempts to modify problems in the care of the hospitalized patient. She should be aware of the role that anxiety plays in causing the patient to regress and become dependent. She can, with observation, become cognizant of the relationship between anxiety and pain. The nurse who wants to understand the patient's needs must be aware of explicit, implicit, rational, irrational, and symbolic patterns of behavior.

Anxiety is a vague but nonetheless persistent feeling of discomfort. It has been defined as the psychological response of the human being to *internal* danger. This is in contradistinction to fear, which is the psychological and physical response to *external* danger. The definition implies that the object of anxiety cannot be readily identified; that of fear is recognized easily. Anxiety is the response to an intrapsychic value that is endangered. Fear is a response to physical danger.

The hospitalized patient is bombarded by physical and psychological stresses. He responds to these with anxiety. This diffuse feeling of discomfort can run the gamut from mild sensations of restlessness and butterflies in the stomach to intense discomfort, with agitation or even panic. The patient's behavior will be markedly influenced by the degree of anxiety he experiences. One can look upon the behavior of an anxious patient as an attempt to alleviate his discomfort.

The patient is like a pressure cooker. As long as anxiety is at a comfortable level, the patient will be reasonably serene. If the patient has a means of funneling off increased anxiety, like the valve on a pressure cooker, he can maintain his equilibrium. If there is no escape valve for the steam (which is like the patient's anxiety), the pressure cooker either explodes or the steam seeps out from under the lid of the cooker. So it is that the patient who feels intense discomfort from anxiety either reflects it in his behavior or develops a severe psychological or physiological diathesis. Two modes of behavior that may develop from the pressure of anxiety are regression and dependency.

Being an advocate of the patient is a grave responsibility. When that patient is regressed and dependent, the responsibility is even greater, since the nurse must contend not only with the transmission of information but with a mode of communication that is effective through the malignant obstruction of stress, anxiety, and misfortune. To communicate anything—be it information, attitude, or sensitivity—it is necessary to understand and use appropriate communication modalities. Fundamentally, the task is to send a message in such a way that the respondent can interpret it correctly and respond to it. Thus, the message *sender* must decide what he wishes to communicate. He must put the message into language that the respondent (receiver) will understand; in other words, he must *encode* it. The communication cycle is not complete until the respondent *decodes* the message and indicates his understanding by offering appropriate *feedback* to the sender.

In the case of communication between nurse and patient, several factors operate to the detriment of the completed communication cycle:

1. Both parties have certain assumptions concerning the meaning of the other's messages based upon their perceptions of the other's identity. This, in turn, is colored by the *roles* assumed by both. It is

often difficult to make one's point as a caring human being when the person is accepted as a "sterile, starched nurse."

2. Messages often must be decoded under the influence of such stresses as pain, fear, and lack of time. These factors may distort the meaning of the communication. If, for instance, a patient is on call to the operating room and the call is received to prepare the patient to be picked up immediately, the nurse is likely to rush into the patient's room, blurt out that the operating room has called, medicate the patient, gown him, and be barely finished when the attendant arrives with a stretcher. In such a situation, the patient is hardly able to describe his feelings nor is the nurse able to act as the patient's advocate, explaining, preparing, easing, and caring.

3. Messages may be distorted by events that have transpired between nurse and patient in the past or those that will occur in the future. If, for instance, the nurse must administer intramuscular medication in oil suspension b.i.d. and liver extract, and she must subject the patient to painful treatments, that patient is likely to come to resent her. It is not enough that the nurse does these things to enable the patient to recover. He aches *now*. The nebulous future is of little moment in terms of his black and blue buttocks, or in terms of his dread as he hears his door open each morning when he knows these events will occur. Such a patient has been conditioned to respond in a given manner, and it influences the communication cycle.

The effective nurse who truly cares that her patient hears and understands her must listen to the kinds of words her patient uses. Does he say the painful nights are "pretty tough"? Does the gynecologic patient talk about her "fire balls"? In the latter case, the nurse will be more effective in explaining to the patient about her disease process if she too uses the words "fire balls" rather than fibroids. For the patient who describes his anxiety attacks as attacks of "nerves," the nurse needs to respond in like terminology.

It is better to use descriptive words rather than interpretative labels. How does "anxious" feel? What is it like to have an "attack of nerves"? Is the patient frightened? If so, of what? When nurse and patient can filter their communications down to specifics, they can sometimes attenuate feelings such as fear or anger or sadness by altering the forces responsible for these feelings.

A word may be used by the patient that has an entirely different connotation for the nurse. What of the patient who speaks of his possible "growth"? To the nurse, such a word may mean a tumor, benign or malignant. For the patient, "growth" may mean cancer. The patient may speak of a diagnosed meningioma. To the nurse this means a very low-grade tumor which is usually operable. The patient may be describing an illness which he understands to be a cancerous brain tumor from which he expects to die quite soon. It is necessary to know that sender and receiver of the message mean the same thing in the words they use to encode and decode the messages.

The nurse must put her message in words that the patient will understand. She can do this only by studying the patient's communication techniques well enough to know how the patient himself would transmit a similar message. This done, the nurse awaits feedback from the patient indicating that he has understood the message. Feedback may be an appropriate action such as rolling over or swallowing medication. It may be questions generated by the nurse's statement. It may be a nonverbal communication such as squeezing the nurse's hand, a sudden increase in respiration, or even laughter.

The nurse who desires to be the patient's advocate must be sure that she understands the patient's message. Should she doubt his meaning at all, she must seek clarification. It is not awkward to say, "I'm not sure I understand," or "Can you tell me a little more about that?" Only in this way can nurse and patient obtain a better, more real understanding of one another.

As the patient's advocate, the nurse tries to assist him in his battle against disease, pain, and the anxiety engendered by them. As has been mentioned, pain is an experience that promotes isolation and a feeling of helplessness. These feelings engender anxiety because the patient is concerned about his lack of control of the discomfort. In turn, the anxiety generates greater pain. Thus, a vicious cycle is established. Pain is felt; relief is not forthcoming; anxiety magnifies further pain.

If it is known that the patient is in pain, giving an analgesic before it is requested can be most beneficial. This small courtesy permits the patient greater dignity. He does not have to request that which is rightfully his. These kinds of gestures are translated by the patient as positive feelings toward him. He will understand them as such. The nurse—the mother surrogate, the recipient of the patient's strivings for dependency—will be aiding the patient in a therapeutic manner.

Anxiety is a factor in rational and irrational behavior. It influences explicit behavioral patterns as well as their implicit meanings. Anxiety is even a component of symbolism in patterns of behavior. A central focus in the implementation of one's advocacy of the patient should be sensitivity to his anxiety and its alleviation. A specific approach to this process involves the nurse's communication to her patient that she is a humane, *caring* person. Illness increases the need to be loved and cared for. Enforced inactivity adds to the wish to return to a dependent, more childlike status. The nurse can offer the warmth and caring the patient so desperately needs in a variety of ways. She shows her concern by accepting the patient as he presents himself. His behavior might be difficult to understand at times, but a nonjudgmental handling of it is a way of expressing acceptance of the patient.

The patient's advocate cares. A way to show concern, which is a sign of caring, is to permit and encourage the patient to express himself. Expression is encouraged when the nurse questions the patient in such a manner that he must answer descriptively, rather than in terms of no or yes. When the patient seems comfortable discussing his thoughts and feelings, the nurse might theorize as to how the patient feels and ask him for validation. Taking time to sit with a patient for even a short time is indicative of interest in the individual.

Meeting the sick person's psychological needs in a constructive manner will aid him in reintegrating more mature levels of behavior and will permit him to convalesce and leave the hospital rehabilitated.

BIBLIOGRAPHY

ORLANDO, I: *The Dynamic Nurse-Patient Relationship*. GP Putnam's Sons, New York, 1961.

ROBINSON, L: *Liaison Nursing: A Psychological Approach to Patient Care*. FA Davis, Philadelphia, 1974.

ROBINSON, L: *Psychiatric Nursing as a Human Experience*. WB Saunders, Philadelphia, 1972.

TRAVELBEE, J: *Intervention in Psychiatric Nursing*. FA Davis, Philadelphia, 1968.

Glossary

Anlage. A foundation or rudiment. Parental guidance provides a partial basis for each adult's behavior; the guidance that influences later thinking and behavior may be termed the *anlages* of that behavior.

Anxiety. A feeling of discomfort; can be vague or very intense. Is derived from energy arising from intrapsychic conflict. Associated with internal dangers, that is, threats to self-image or defined values.

Compensation. A defense mechanism in which an approved character trait is emphasized to conceal from the ego the existence of a less desirable one.

Covert. Hidden, as in *covert* message; that part of a communication not consciously expressed.

Denial. A defense mechanism; an unconscious process which permits the individual to be unaware of that which is too stressful for his ego.

Depressive equivalent. A physical symptom or syndrome that masks the patient's underlying depression. As long as the patient feels the physical symptom, he is unaware of his depression.

Fantasy. A psychic mechanism that occurs when the individual is awake, like a daydream. Is readily made conscious when the individual is requested to be introspective and focus on his thoughts. It is a normal process, but excessive use enables the individual to escape from reality into his less harsh dream world. An extreme degree of fantasying is related to psychosis. Young children fantasy extensively in their play.

Genital strivings. Are related to a developmental phase and describe the individual's level of performance. The individual who has reached maturity psychosexually is able to relate to others in a productive manner; the term *genital strivings* implies that that individual has reached sexual maturation.

Heterosexual. An individual who is able to and prefers to relate to members of opposite sex; one whose development has progressed beyond the chumship level of puberty.

Homosexual. An individual who prefers to relate to members of his or her own sex, who may or may not be perceived as love objects.

Identification. An unconscious mechanism by which an individual conceives of himself as similar to an admired person. May involve copying external features, such as clothes.

Identity. Self-image or self-concept. Has its initial development in the definition of body image, but subsequently includes percepts of self related to a set of values, an armamentarium of strength, weaknesses, and skills, a sex *identity*, a repertory of social roles, internalized relationships with a number of territorial objects, and membership status in a variety of groups. This information is absolutely necessary to enable the self to run the maze of social relationships, and seems to be most efficiently acquired through social interaction.

Latent. Hidden, potential.

Narcissism. Love of self. Term derived from Greek myth about Narcissus, who fell in love with his own image reflected in a pool of water. A normal self-preservative emotion, but is pathological when experienced to such a degree that other relationships, emotions, and love objects are denied importance.

Overt. Open, conscious.

Pregenital. A term descriptive of a phase of psychosexual development. The *pregenital* personality is sexually immature; interests are directed at an earlier developmental level. The individual is not motivated to develop one-to-one heterosexual relationships.

Projection. A mental mechanism that buffers the ego by unconsciously attributing one's own displeasing thoughts or feelings to others, such as a person who hates someone and thinks that that person hates him. This mechanism is used extensively by psychotic people who feel persecuted.

Regression. A mental mechanism in which the individual operates on an earlier level of development in order to help the ego withstand stress (anxiety). Can be useful and nonpathological for the physically ill patient, or can be a symptom of severe mental illness, as in the schizophrenic patient who remains in one position constantly, is mute, and soils.

Repression. An unconscious mechanism in which one keeps thoughts, feelings, and perceptions in the unconscious in order to shield the ego from stresses it cannot tolerate, such as an adult male's inability to remember the character of his love (sexual attraction) for his mother during the oedipal phase of development.

Self-image. *See* Identity.

Set. The attitude or interest of an observer that may influence his perception, such as a person who feels fat or unattractive perceiving these qualities when he sees his reflection in a mirror.

Sexuality. The nature of an individual in relation to sexual attitudes or activity.

System. A bounded territory in space and time. Input and output processes occur over the boundaries. Passage of information or signals from one individual organism to another has been studied as a communication process. Ion exchange across a cell membrane, passage of nutrients through the lining of the intestine, and respiratory exchange in the alveoli of the lungs are well-studied examples.

Index

A page number in italics indicates an illustration; a page number followed by *t* indicates a table.